ADVANCE PRAISE FOR
DAN ISAACSON AND *THE EQUATION*

"Lisa and I can both attest to the fact that The Equation works. The results are clear and absolute, and have given us simple, yet profound changes and amazing results. This book should be the 'How To' manual for life."
—*Clint Black (and Lisa Hartman)*

"Dan helps me with everything. Instead of eating a little bit for dinner, he will have me eat five small meals during the day so you always feel like you are getting something. You don't feel deprived." —*Billy Crystal*

"Dan sets the standard in fitness for all to follow. He knows the secrets and they work!" —*Rick Dees*

"Dan's work is incredibly generous. . . . He gives you the knowledge and, more important, the desire and courage to approach life and health in a totally different way. I have never felt physically (and as a result of that, spiritually) better in my life than when I worked with Dan or am applying his methods myself. He changed the way I woke up—slept—and everything in between." —*Johnny Depp*

"I've known Dan a long time. He has taught me just about everything I know about health and fitness. Dan inspired me to get into shape early on in my life and he continues to inspire me today." —*Melissa Gilbert*

"I've learned time and again that doing what Dan Isaacson tells you to do results in the loss of pound after pound." —*Tom Hanks*

"Dan—you are the man! An inspiration and simply the best—you got me in great shape many years ago during *Knight Rider* and I've taken your formula with me for years. It works!" —*David Hasselhoff*

"There are certain things that Dan taught me that I am able to incorporate into my own workout schedule that I use to this day." —*Marilu Henner*

"I've had the privilege of knowing Danny since our college fraternity days. He has always demonstrated an unyielding integrity and passion for fitness and health, both of the body and mind, for men and women of all ages. His current book certainly is a reflection of his many years of proof-positive results. I hope you enjoy it as much as I did."
—*Robert Nardelli, President and CEO, The Home Depot*

THE
EQUATION

THE
EQUATION

A 5-Step Program for Lifelong Fitness

Dan Isaacson

with

Dr. Greg Payne *and* Mark Laska

ST. MARTIN'S PRESS · NEW YORK

www.stmartins.com

Library of Congress Cataloging-in-Publication Data

Isaacson, Dan.
    The equation : a 5-step program for lifelong fitness /
Dan Isaacson, with Greg Payne and Mark Laska; foreword by Billy Crystal.
        p. cm.
    ISBN 0-312-28296-6
    1. Weight loss. 2. Nutrition. 3. Exercise. I. Payne, Gregory. II. Laska, Mark. III. Title.

    RM222.2 .I825 2002
    613.7—dc21

                                                    2001058851

First Edition: May 2002

10   9   8   7   6   5   4   3   2   1

CONTENTS

SPECIAL THANKS

Above all, we would like to thank you, the reader, for your bravery. In picking up this book, perusing its contents, and by taking it into your heart, mind, and lifestyle, you are taking a leap of faith to improve your life. We thank you for your confidence, for your efforts, and for allowing us to bring you this information.

Our deepest thanks to St. Martin's Press, especially Heather Jackson-Silverman, for being the most thoughtful and thorough editor of all time. Our gratitude to Mel Berger, for being an unyielding pillar of integrity, and always making it work out. Special thanks to Rick Hersh and the rest of the William Morris family: without you this would never have been possible. We also would like to express our indebtedness to all medical, research, academic, and fitness professionals whose vigilance and dedication enrich the lives of the many—you are heroes all. Thanks to the Hollywood community for their openness and support: you have led others to live a healthy lifestyle by your example. Last but not least, heartfelt thanks to our friends and family for your contributions, patience, support, and understanding.

AUTHOR'S NOTE

This book suggests a reasonable approach to realistic weight loss. Before implementing any of the suggestions contained within this book, please consult with your doctor. While we believe that this book reflects information that has been widely accepted by the medical, research, and academic communities, please bring this book to his or her attention so that you can have professional assurance that the methodologies contained herein are correct for your personal use.

In 1995, the U.S. Surgeon General issued an incredibly dramatic report. Contained in this report was the most groundbreaking information ever conveyed to the public regarding the importance of exercise. For the first time, the Surgeon General linked inactivity and being overweight to the most threatening diseases and greatest killers known to man. The Centers for Disease Control stated in no uncertain terms that inactivity and poor eating habits were responsible for as many deaths per year as smoking-related diseases. The medical, research, academic, and fitness communities rejoiced in these pro-active statements, expecting that finally Americans would plainly see that to become leaner and more fit could mean many extra years and far less suffering from debilitating illnesses. To our amazement and disappointment this message went unheard. In the years that have followed, the National Institutes of Health, the Centers for Disease Control, and the American Medical Association have all attempted to reinforce or rephrase the contents of the Surgeon General's report. All have been met with the same reaction. For some reason, few understood the ramifications of these important findings. It seems to us that the problem isn't with the information . . . the problem is that people do not know how to use the information.

This book was written to convey the information contained within the Surgeon General's report, and to provide you with a format so that you can implement and benefit from the scientific findings compiled by the National Institutes of Health, the Centers for Disease Control, and the American Medical Association. This book combines everything that has been scientifically proven to work with simple and effective methods to utilize that information. By using that information not only will you become leaner and more fit, but you may also add many years to your life and have the greatest opportunity to live those years with vitality and without disease.

FOREWORD

I was never good in math, but the proof for this Equation is it works. I have worked with Dan Isaacson for almost sixteen years. He has trained me for movies, press junkets, and other events. Usually, we have six to eight weeks and a deadline to hone in on. Now, our workouts have a different goal, plain old staying in shape gets harder and harder as we get older. Yes, even I am aging.

What Dan has done over the years is to constantly study ways to make working out fun and effective. But that's only part of the project. You can pump all the iron you want, but if you're also pumping cake, it just won't work. He is always trying to figure out the best way for anyone to maintain a level of fitness through diet and exercise.

I have tried everything, and The Equation is the best. You can't assume because you're lifting and working out that all will fall into place, or rather off the places, you want to lose weight. It's a combination of so many things. Sooner or later, we all have to change our way of doing things.

The Equation that this book gives us is the best one for me. I know, you can say, "Billy's not a big guy, he doesn't have a problem, what's he talking about?" Believe me, I can inflate too. And my energy levels are crucial to me, especially if I'm making a film.

This book is not a trick or a gimmick: it's a very easy-to-follow way of life. I never feel that I'm depriving myself, or this is torture. Once you get it into your head, which is the most important muscle to flex, that things have to be different, then just follow The Equation, and I know you'll get the same results I have.

—*Billy Crystal*

INTRODUCTION

You already know that The Equation works. You see the results of this program every time you turn on the television or go to the movies. The most dramatic physical transformations in Hollywood history have been achieved by using The Equation, and now you can use the exact same program.

The Equation is not a radical approach. It doesn't limit your choices, or make you starve yourself. The Equation combines all of the information that exists on losing fat, weight, and inches, and teaches you how to use that information to reach your goal.

The authors of this book have been leaders in making cutting-edge medical information applicable in people's everyday lives. To many, Dan Isaacson is the original "trainer to the stars" and a true pioneer of the personal training movement. He has been behind the highest-profile celebrity transformations over the last twenty years. Dr. Greg Payne is the chair of the Department of Human Performance at San Jose State University and is one of the nation's foremost experts on exercise and obesity. Isaacson and Payne met while serving on the California Governor's Council on Physical Fitness. This organization takes information compiled by the Surgeon General, Centers for Disease Control, and other front-line institutions, and promotes programs on the state and local levels so that the greatest number of people can benefit from and utilize that information. In much the same way, this book has been written to provide you with the most up-to-date and scientifically sound information concerning weight loss, and combines it with a practical methodology so that you can apply that information to your own personal transformation.

If you could take all of the information that exists on dieting and nutrition, all the information that exists on exercise and fitness and distill it down to what has been scientifically proven to work, you would be left with The Equation. Everyone who has lost weight or inches essentially does the exact same thing. No matter what the name of their diet, no matter what kind of exercise they used, they all did many similar things to achieve their transformation. This common ground is The Equation, and everyone you know who has ever lost weight and inches has used The Equation to get those results.

The beauty of The Equation is in its simplicity. Without doubt, this is the easiest and most effective program that you will ever come across. There is no gimmick. There is no potion, pill, or powder. Your success comes from making the smallest, most painless, and almost imperceptible adjustments to your daily life. Each week you layer in another tiny adjustment into your daily routine. When combined, these adjustments will have a dramatic effect on the way you look and feel, get you results in the quickest possible time, and allow you to keep the results you achieve for the rest of your life.

The Equation is about transforming your lifestyle and, by doing so, transforming your physical appearance. The Equation is a road map to get there—a step-by-step guidebook to improve your health and appearance forever. By simply turning the page you will begin to change your life for the better.

EQUATION

for

CHANGE

You wouldn't be reading this book if you didn't want to change your weight or your appearance or improve some other aspect of your life. The dictionary defines *change* as "to make different in form or to transform." This book is all about change.

Change can occur on both a large and a small scale. Look at any sport to find an example. A team comes in last place one season, rebuilds the team in the off-season, and is competitive the next season. It was not because of one player. The team filled its roster with different role players, each of them with his own specialty. If those specialties are complementary to one another, the team becomes a winner. For an amateur tennis player to turn professional, every aspect of her game has to be outstanding. If her backhand, forehand, or net game is weak, chances are she won't be able to compensate for the deficiency and make up for it with a great overhead smash. One ball in the net, another ball out, and she cannot be competitive. So she works on the aspect of her game that is weak. In 1985, Dan trained a driver competing in the Indy 500. For the entire month of May that year, the Penske team made slight adjustments to Danny Sullivan's car. They adjusted the airfoil slightly, they tinkered with different brands of tires, they adjusted the torque slightly, they fiddled with the fuel injection until everything on the car ran perfectly. During the race, they made slight adjustments during each of the 200 laps. Danny Sullivan won the Indy 500 that year with what is considered to be one of the most exciting finishes of all time. Small changes won the race. A big change to either the tires or the airfoil or any other part of the car, or the way he was driving it, would have lost the race for him.

The point is that any big change you make or think about making can happen only if it is supported by smaller changes. So if you want a big change result, like going from last to first place, the key is small changes over time.

Everything starts with having a vision of the big change and then committing to a process or strategy that will enable you to effect that big change. Your strategy consists of small changes that you can implement on a daily basis. The big change we are talking about in this book is a physical transformation. A physical transformation, no matter how big or small, no matter what your age or level of physical ability, utilizes the same exact concepts and principles for success. Those principles will consistently be the small changes you make every day, and maintaining those changes over time. This is the secret of success: To make a big change in your physical appearance, you will need a specific game plan. Each chapter in the book will make a suggestion of one small change to incorporate into your normal daily behavior.

If physical transformation is your goal, perhaps the first thing you could and should ponder is what you are currently doing in the course of the day, looking specifically at what you are eating. Do you have any habits or preferences that might prevent you from looking the way would like to look? If and when you can identify these stumbling blocks, you can go about dealing with them appropriately. These obstacles to success can be overcome, and to achieve the results you want, it is essential that these obstacles be eliminated. For every obstacle that you face, you can always get around it by employing three different options. The most appropriate alternatives to any obstacle are to substitute, modify, or shift.

SUBSTITUTE, MODIFY, AND SHIFT

Substitute, modify, and shift are the three keys to realizing the big change you have envisioned. These are three separate strategies that will allow you to adhere to any given strategy, and they are the three methods to defeat any obstacle that stands in the way of your goal.

Perhaps you eat ice cream every night before you go to bed. To effect the change you are seeking, you'll probably have to alter this habit. To alter this habit, to overcome this obstacle, you have three basic choices. First, you can *substitute* healthy foods in place of what you know is keeping you from reaching your goal. Your second option is to *modify* or to eat half of the food that keeps you from achieving your goal. That will certainly reduce a part of the problem. Your third option is to *shift* what you are doing. To shift, you may decide on a different time to eat your ice cream. If you allowed yourself ice cream only before 10 A.M., chances are you wouldn't have any. By implementing any of these three strategies—substitute, modify, and shift—you can and will effect the larger change. The most effective options for that particular example follow in this order: Substitution is the best solution. Substituting healthy foods for the foods you know are full of sugar and saturated fat will definitely improve your weight-loss potential and your overall health. Modifying the amount of food you eat is still a pathway to improvement, so obviously if you eat less of it, you are on the right track. Finally, the most difficult strategy is to shift the circumstances of that obstacle or otherwise dramatically alter your behavior patterns. To shift implies a sweeping change like going from the activity level of a barnacle to the fitness regimen of an Olympic athlete. However, if you could actually accommodate that shift and maintain it, the results would be magnificent.

Change is not easy. As human beings we are a tremendously adaptable species, capable of surviving almost any climate or calamity, and yet we are creatures of habit and those habits are not changed easily. But change is exactly what is required for you to alter your weight or your appearance, or to improve any other aspect of your life.

Change and *results* are not the same thing. It will take patience to reach your ideal goal. Small changes bring about results over time. It is worth repeating: *Small changes bring about results over time.* Finally we have to remember that while small changes bring about results, any results you do achieve will be limited to what you have been given. If you are five-three and big boned, nothing will make you five-six and willowy. It just can't happen. When you envision the ideal physique for yourself, it is essential that you acknowledge that you have your body to work with. Just like the automakers of our world, we have a body style. Some of us have metabolic rates, muscle fiber, and fat storage capabilities that act like a sports car. Others have the more standard two-door or four-door sedan, while still others have bodies that more closely resemble an SUV. We all have different shapes and sizes. That does not mean that you cannot make changes to the engine to make it run better or make it more gas efficient, or keep the repairs up so you have fewer hefty bills with your automobile. Furthermore, you can change the look and value of your own car by how well you take care of it. It is up to you how you want to look and how you want to feel. Line up all these cars in a row and they all look hot and sexy, each has a specific function, and they are all appealing in their own way.

Behavioral scientists and experts agree that there are five stages to change.[1] Step One is called pre-contemplation. In this phase you are not even thinking about a change or are even cognizant that a change needs to be made. Pat yourself on the back, because by even opening up this book you have bypassed this stage and started the process of change. The Equation will guide you through five stages that will help you make small changes that produce amazing results. 1. Pre-Contemplative, 2. The Contemplative Stage, 3. The Action Stage, 4. The Goal-Oriented Action Stage, and 5. The Maintenance Stage. This book is separated into five parts to guide you through the process of making a change, getting the results you desire, personalizing the equation to meet goals, and maintaining those results for the rest of your life.

You have gone past the first stage of your physical transformation, and are now in the contemplative stage. At this moment, you are beginning to think about effecting a change in your appearance and the composition of your body. This stage is a bit like dipping your toes in the water to test the temperature before jumping in. Testing the water requires the decision to stick your toes in the water, and dipping your toes in thereafter is not the same as doing nothing. To the contrary, thinking about what you want to change and how you want to effect that change are profound steps. As an experiment, list the changes you want to make and the effects of those changes on your life. First, write down in your own words how you would like to look and feel. In your mind's eye, really get a picture of what you would like to look like. If you did look like that, how would you feel? What would your health be like? What kinds of activities would you or could you participate in that you are not currently doing? What would your sex life be like? How would you feel about yourself? Would you be more confident? Would you feel more comfortable? What would be the difference in your wardrobe? Would you relate to others differently? Now you must contemplate how you would like to make those changes happen.

Much like any other big decision you have to face, you are doing your research, you are discovering what options are available to you, and you are trying to determine what course of action to pursue. This information will be extremely valuable to you in the long run and will enable you to get from point A to point B. Spending the time contemplating how to reach your destination can certainly mean the difference between success and failure when it comes to creating the ideal nutritional and activity program for yourself. In this stage, you are mentally weighing your prospects. Take the time to determine what is best for you.

Part One of this book deals exclusively with the issues that are most important to you at this very moment. The chapters in this section discuss the ins and outs of dieting, what works and what doesn't. Gradually, the first part of this book will move you into the next phase of your transformation, the phase called action, when you really do something about the situation you would like to change.

CHAPTER ONE

Contemplating Change

They say that timing is everything. You are incredibly lucky. Your timing is perfect.

You want to change your body. You want to drop some weight. You want to look leaner. You want to become more fit and healthy. Well, you couldn't have chosen a better time. Obviously, sooner is always better than later to make this change. However, your timing is perfect because we know much more about losing weight than at any other time in history. There have been so many people who have made a similar journey. There have been so many trailblazers, so many pioneers, so many innovators, and so many people who have experimented with losing weight, that your journey today is less treacherous and hazardous. It is because of their failures and successes that your journey will be simple and easy. It is because of their failures and their successes that you have the benefit of an abundance of information and knowledge. Not all of this information may be helpful. Not all of this knowledge may be scientifically sound. As a result, not all of this information is worth your time. Most of this information does not make good common sense. Even less of this information will actually work for you. From decades of trial, error, and application, we can show you what has been proven to work and how to use this information.

Contemplation is something we all do all the time. Most of us, however, do not go through the process systematically. If you want to contemplate any change, you must answer five questions. Identify and think about the following during the contemplative stage:

1. What do I want to do?
2. How do I want to do it?
3. What will it cost?
4. How much time will it take?
5. How will it affect my family and work responsibilities?

Every individual will have different answers, and every person has a different level of commitment. Answering these questions will help you start putting together a format that you can live with and will begin the customization process of what you will do and what you won't do. The process of going through the contemplative stage really helps you prepare for action. Unless you are fully prepared for and committed to the process we've just noted, and know the answers to each of those questions, then you'll never really be able to make the action phase happen. It is a very important phase.

The idea behind this book is not to prescribe one specific, certain way to lose weight. That is a flawed approach. Thousands of different diets exist, and there are many philosophies about how to lose weight. The Equation separates the wheat from the chaff and encapsulates the information that has been scientifically proven to work. This book represents an easy-to-use guide that shows you what all *the plans that do work* have in common. This book represents all the hard, cold facts that link all the various philosophies that have helped people succeed. It is a step-by-step guide that will enable you to layer these philosophies and habits into your own life and make them fit within your lifestyle. In short, we provide all the information you need to be successful in losing fat and weight, and teach you how to use that information. In fact, The Equation is not a fad diet. In fact, The Equation is not even a "diet." The Equation is not a gimmick. The Equation is about making small, easy-to-accomplish adjustments to your lifestyle, holding on to these new adjustments for the rest of your life, and allowing those minor adjustments to transform the way you look and feel—forever.

The Equation is a simple concept to convey. Losing weight is simple: eat less and move more. Everyone you know who has lost weight has done one or the other or both. You could comprehend all of the information contained in this book in a very short time, but it is one thing to understand what it means to you and another for the information to be useful. We could explain each part of your automobile, how that part connects with all the other parts, and all the advantages of the internal combustion engine, but wouldn't you just rather have the keys and drive it? We wrote this book so that you can begin using and benefiting from this information immediately. Just turn it on and you are on your way. No matter what speed you choose to drive, you will always be on the right road.

CHAPTER TWO

The Human Laboratory

We are all unique. A nutritional program that works for me may not work for you. What may have worked for your mother, your father, your brother, or your sister, despite all of their physiological similarities, may not be the answer for you. Whatever worked for you five years ago might not even work for you today. To have success, you have to assume the mind-set of an explorer or an inventor or a scientist. This is a journey; a combination of different items that make something entirely new and functional; a grand experiment that must be proven to work. You are extremely fortunate that much of the experimentation has already been done for you.

YOUR PERSONAL EXPERIMENT

To make a physical transformation, you have a whole world of options available to you. There are so many different strategies you could employ. There are so many ways you could alter each of these strategies. There are so many traps you could fall into along the way that could block you from your goal. The Equation gives focus to your experiment and distills the world of possibilities down to only what works. It is much like narrowing 360 degrees of vision to about 20 degrees. Within the confines of the 20 degrees that has been proven to work, your experimentation will be limited to what works for you personally. Much of this experimentation depends on what you will do and what you will not do, what you are capable of doing and what you are incapable of doing for the rest of your life.

SUCCESSFUL EXPERIMENTS–
THE HISTORY OF HEALTH AND FITNESS

People study history so they won't repeat the mistakes of the past, and you should look at losing fat, weight, and inches in much the same way. There are definite historical landmarks that should be followed and many more that should be avoided. When studying the history of dieting, weight loss, and exercise, you will find that athletes have performed the vast majority of experimentation. These athletes provide a perfect example, because they were both the "scientist" performing the experiment and, like you, they were also their own subject or "guinea pig."

People have been concerned about their physiques for a long time. The ancient Greeks started this whole obsession when they began to ponder the ideal human body. It is believed that the ancient Greeks were the first to employ strength training as a means to transform their bodies when a young man started lifting a calf several times every day, and by the time the calf became a steer, the young man had much larger muscles. In ancient Greek society, physical training was done largely to become more adept in warfare, however, they also practiced sport. In addition to strength training, the Greeks began a number of competitive sporting events, which, of course, eventually evolved into what we know as the Olympics. It can be assumed with some certainty that they noticed that strenuous exercise had a direct effect on the physique. The ancient Romans also idealized the perfect human body and were obsessed with improving upon their own. The Romans were much more concerned with sport than even the Greeks, and it was the Romans who gave us the notion of health clubs and what we now know as weight training.

No real groundbreaking improvements were made to sports, aerobic training, or strength training until the 1800s. During the 1800s, the Olympics were revived as a peaceful competition among nations, and this marked a renewal of interest in physical activity. At this point, people, mostly men, began training for these events and noticed again that with exercise came a certain level of leanness, virility, and health. At the time, obesity was not a major concern, but most desperately wanted to be healthier in order to live longer. Several wealthy businessmen opened up retreat centers in the late 1800s and early 1900s that catered to the wealthy. At these retreat centers, numerous therapeutic procedures were available, along with regular exercise and nutritional advice. Depicted in novels such as *The Road to Wellville* (also later made into a film with Anthony Hopkins and Matthew Broderick), these retreat centers were generally regarded as sham organizations, pseudoscientific havens for charlatans. Although this marked the first time that nutritional guidelines were given to patients, and proper nutrition and exercise were linked as a strategy to combat excess fat and to promote optimum health, their methods were crude and primitive.

As if shamed into oblivion, exercise and nutrition fell by the wayside and were not a subject of interest to anyone except athletes and performers, at least not until the 1950s. Nutrition and exercise were viewed differently by each of the sexes. For boys and young men of every economic level, there were sports, sports, and more sports. As men grew into adulthood and reached a certain level of affluence, there were country clubs and gentlemen's clubs where business deals were made over a game of golf, a game of squash, or in the steam room. For girls and young women, most exercise centered around some form of dance. Then television changed everything. In the 1950s, Jack LaLanne, a world champion bodybuilder and athlete, came into our living rooms and changed the way everyone regarded exercise and nutrition. At the beginning of each show, LaLanne would give a short pep talk and a nutrition tip, and then would do a workout that progressed through every major muscle group in the body. He called his system of exercises "Trimnastics."

EXERCISE AND NUTRITION

Until this point, exercise and nutrition had been two different worlds of study, two different and separate strategies that had no relationship with one another. In an instant, all of that changed. Who really knows why? It might have been the newness or the reach of television. It may have been that people were just ready to hear the information. It may have been that the messenger was so passionate, so knowledgeable, and so devoted to the message. It may have been because he was and is a living example of what proper nutrition and exercise can actually do for your body and for your spirit. Perhaps he was just the first genuine fitness role model. In any case, Jack LaLanne has been passionately teaching us about exercise and nutrition for more than fifty years. He has done so much to bring useful, pertinent, lifesaving, and life-prolonging information into our common consciousness. Without him, the right person at the right time, these messages might not have had the same impact. To this day, LaLanne continues to inspire and teach us about exercise and nutrition and the benefits they offer at every stage in life.

His accomplishments are countless. But the greatest gifts he gave to each passing generation were to inextricably link nutrition with exercise and prove to us that with the proper combination of both, we could change our bodies, our mental outlooks, and our lives.

THE EXERCISE REVOLUTION

Many have come since and added to the knowledge he shared with us. In the 1950s, Bonnie Prudden noticed a change in the physical education curriculum of her two young daughters. Rather than engaging in rigorous physical activity, the activity had shifted to play activities and games. Watching her children become less and less active, she began a conditioning class and developed a dance-based exercise program that enabled children to become more physically fit. Brought to the attention of Dwight D. Eisenhower this work led to the formation of the President's Council on Physical Fitness and Sports, and to the mandatory inclusion of physical fitness into the curriculum of students nationwide.

Numerous others have contributed to the field of fitness. One of the more prominent was Dr. Thomas K. Cureton, who through the University of Illinois Physical Fitness Research Laboratory not only developed a new system of training but also taught and mentored almost all of the leaders in this field. Cureton developed and wrote the *Physical Fitness Workbook,* which was used by Y's, the military, schools, and colleges around the country. This program was the precursor of what we now know as aerobics, step aerobics, and cardiovascular interval training. This program inspired the Royal Canadian Air Force Exercises, which inspired the U.S. Air Force "Aerobics" Program, which was designed by Lt. Col. Ken Cooper.

With this landmark work, the medical establishment began to give credence to the role of exercise in the treatment and prevention of cardiovascular disease and obesity. Scholarly research was starting to emerge from a handful of university programs, and this laid the foundation for a scientific body of knowledge relating to exercise and health. The American College of Sports Medicine became very active in disseminating information to the medical community and provided convincing proof that there was a scientific basis that linked exercise with health and the efficiency of the heart and cardiovascular system. This scientific basis was so sound that not only was it embraced and instituted by the medical community, but now exercise and nutritional guidelines are put out by the U.S. Department of Health and Human Services as well as the Centers for Disease Control and Prevention.

HOW DOES HISTORY APPLY TO
MY PHYSICAL TRANSFORMATION?

In the 1960s and 1970s there were many who contributed to the vast amount of information you will need and use for your own physical transformation. Again, most of this information came by way of athletes, and the information on physical transformation is mostly within the context of exercise. These athletes, while trying to improve their performance, happened to create some wonderful answers to the questions we all have, and they came upon those answers mostly by accident. These successful accidents were carefully noted and applied by other athletes and observant coaches, who were able to pass them along to other athletes and refine the process to improve results for the next athlete. Soon, these people became exalted figures because of what they could deliver.

One of the great examples of athletic experimentation turning into literal gold was Olympian Frank Shorter. After becoming the first American marathon runner to win the gold medal in the 1972 games, he brought jogging to the forefront of the American psyche. Jim Fixx and his book *The Complete Book of Running* brought this message to corporate America, and soon executives across the nation found that by exercising regularly they not only became more lean but also more productive in the office. The jogging craze led to the tennis craze, which led to the aerobics craze, which led to the gym craze. When the gym craze began, it seemed that the entire country was working out and dieting to look their best. One fad was quickly replaced by the next, and most people were blindly chasing the elusive thing that would get them the results they were so desperate for.

SO WHAT HAPPENED TO US?

If you're reading this book you've probably decided you need to lose a few—or more—pounds of fat. You might have wondered over the years whatever happened to that svelte body of yours. If you're like many Americans, you were relatively lean at one point, but then over several years or decades, fat, or even obesity, creeped in. You reached a point where you noticed much more fat than you'd like. Well, if this describes you, you're not alone. According to the Centers for Disease Control, the percentage of young people in the United States who are overweight has more than doubled in the last thirty years with nearly 14 percent of children and 12 percent of teens being obese. Children who are obese have an overwhelming chance of being obese forever. Overall, about 50 percent of Americans are overweight and 25 percent of the population could be considered obese. There has been a 2 percent overall increase in percent body fat for all age groups over the last quarter century. Nearly a third of a million people each year die from nutrition and physical inactivity related diseases.[2]

Why all the gloom and doom? Why the explosion in fat weight among Americans? Most experts agree that the answers to these questions are complex. Many factors have contributed to make some astounding societal changes across the past century. Just imagine, we started in the early 1900s as a relatively agrarian society. If we wanted to eat, we had to till the land, nurture it laboriously, then work it again to reap the final benefits of our labor. Manual labor was the norm as we expended substantial energy most days of the week just to exist. However, with increasing industrialization, labor-saving devices became more common; change erupted quickly and dramatically. Imagine the labor-saving devices that evolved over the past century, everything from the car to the automatic dishwasher to the leaf blower. Is it any wonder that many Americans have fallen into a very sedentary lifestyle?

In the middle of the last century we saw the advent of both television and fast food. So while we were sitting more, food became available on demand. It was fast, cheap, and tasty (some would say). It also contained very high levels of fat, making it a major contributor to the most common cause of death in America, heart disease.

In the last quarter century we have seen an even greater technological explosion. In addition to TV, computers are now ever-present. We E-mail rather than walk down the hall to chat with a colleague. Computer games have replaced the game of catch Dad may have had with the kids. And rather than kick-the-can, we now play any number of popular video games. Physical activity has declined dramatically. In short, we have been industrialized, computerized, and supersized into a society that finds itself in an obesity epidemic. Is it any wonder that we are fatter than ever?

EXERCISE WORKS

Through the experience and experimentation of others, we absolutely and positively know that exercise works as a strategy to lose fat, weight, and inches. By increasing your level of activity, you can and will affect the amount of fat on your body. When you expend energy, your body requires fuel for power. This fuel comes from the food you eat. When that is burned off, you still need to power your activity, so your body must find that fuel. Our fat cells act as a fuel storage system. When the food we eat is burned off as fuel for activity, we burn off even more fat by calling upon our fuel storage system. When we tap into this reserve tank, we can reduce the amount of fat on our bodies.

This is effective only to a certain point. If you eat so much that you never tap into your "reserve tank" of fuel, you may never call upon stored fat to power your activity. Exercise can be an effective fat fighter only if it is linked to a sound nutritional program. When you create an effective nutritional plan and combine it with an effective activity strategy, you can structure both to serve your greater purposes. Your greater purpose is to meet your goal. If you can honestly agree that exercise or activity is an effective way to rid yourself of fat, you should now turn your contemplation toward an effective nutritional program.

TAKING A PAGE FROM THE HOLLYWOOD SCRIPT

Most of us know that proper nutrition and exercise will help us to live longer and prevent many diseases. We know, without doubt, that through nutrition and exercise we can have a better quality of life, greater energy, and less stress. Yet many of us would trade all of our good health if only we could be as thin as we would like to be. The process of dieting and exercising is usually not an undertaking that is done for health reasons; people generally do these things to look better. All of us want to look as good as we possibly can. All of us want to be more appealing. All of us want to be more attractive inside and outside of our clothes. In short, dieting is primarily a vanity issue. We want results and we want them yesterday.

Hollywood, as it turns out, provided the bridge that linked what was happening in the world of nutrition with what was happening in the world of exercise. Hollywood is a great example of the exact quandary that most dieters face. Most people want a desired result in a certain amount of time. So it is with actors training for a motion picture. By linking what was considered to be the most cutting-edge information on nutrition with the exercise regimens of athletes, a program was created that could assure physical transformation. This program has been perfected for actors who need to have a certain physical transformation in a certain amount of time. So specific are the goals of these artists that the methods must be precise. In the end, the program boils down to a basic math problem.

The Equation represents this exact math problem. With years of research, with decades of practical application, with thousands of experiments, The Equation uses all we know about how the body functions and rids itself of fat, and uses those natural processes to get exacting results.

The Equation has been proven to work over and over and over again. It has been perfected to such a degree, it is so exact, that your results are guaranteed as surely as $1 + 1 = 2$. Turn on your television or go to the movies and you are likely to see the results with your own eyes. This information, once the exclusive domain of elite athletes and the biggest household names in entertainment, is all here for you to use, and because so much of the experimentation has already been done for you, you can begin to focus on fine-tuning what has already been proven to work. The remainder of this chapter provides a context in which you can begin strategizing your own physical transformation and offers a shortcut for your own experimentation, so that you can create a personalized approach to reach your goals.

When Jack LaLanne first came into our living rooms, we knew that there were two ways to lose weight and trim down: diet and exercise. In all the years since that time, nothing else has been proven to work. During those years we have seen people exercise, and we know that exercise does work to a degree, but really and truly works only in conjunction with the right diet. There is no pill, no powder, no potion, and no magic spell that will help you get the results you want. The only answer is to do more of the activity you are already doing and begin to watch your intake of food. Over the last few pages you have read what exercise has done for others, and that increasing your activity level will work, or at least help in the process of weight loss. But the subject of dieting is still clouded in mystery.

There are many possible answers to the question of "perfect" nutrition. There are many theories about what to do and how to do it. You could literally spend the rest of your life trying this diet and that diet, but in truth, you would probably end up right where you are now, searching for answers. Since we have done so much experimenting with what works and what doesn't, we can limit your focus a little and provide some groundwork for your own experimentation.

DIET IS A FOUR-LETTER WORD

Dieting. Aren't you sick of it? It has become an American obsession. Every time you turn on your television, check your E-mail, or walk through the grocery store checkout line, you are bombarded by the notion of losing weight. There are so many choices and options available that it is almost mind-numbing. We are overwhelmed by empty promises in the form of "Fat Blockers," herbal amphetamines, and other gimmicks that have proven to be fatal to some. We are faced with Weight Watchers, Jenny Craig, Slim-Fast, high-protein diets, high-fat diets, low-fat diets, high carb, no carb, grapefruit diets, cabbage diets, Jamaican diets, Hawaiian diets . . . Where do we turn? There is no filter to separate useful information from charlatanism.

Most of us despise the word *diet*. We despise the word almost as much as going on one, which is definitely an obstacle in itself. The second you think you are going on a diet, you get a large pizza and a gallon of ice cream because, after all, you are starting a diet tomorrow. Diet implies restriction. Diet implies hardship. Diet implies some extreme change from what you are currently doing. Diet implies that you are not beautiful enough, not appealing enough, thin enough, fit enough, and not good enough as you are. Diet implies that you need to be something else or even someone else. Diet is negative. The hard, cold, scientific (and sad) truth is that 99.9 percent of diets do not work in the long term.

WEIGHT LOSS VS. FAT LOSS

The reasons why diets do not work are numerous. The first and most profound reason is that we have lost sight of the real reason we are dieting, and we are trying to change the wrong thing. Just for a moment, forget that your scale exists. How do you know that you need to go on a diet? The next time you get out of the shower, just look at yourself in the bathroom mirror. Now ask yourself, "What needs changing?" Chances are you would want to keep all of your muscle. You certainly cannot live without one or many of your organs. You cannot remove your bones. You could clip your nails and trim your hair, but is that really the weight you want to lose? No! You want to lose the fat. It is the fat you want less of.

Now step on your scale. Does it tell you how much your liver weighs? Does it tell you how much water you have inside your body? Does it tell you how much your bones weigh or how much your muscles weigh? Does it tell you how much your fat weighs? No. Your scale gives you only part of the picture. So when you lose "weight" on your scale, how do you know what you lost? How do you know that you don't just have less water in your system? How do you know that you didn't just lose bone density? How do you know that you lost any fat?

The scale gives you only your total weight, nothing more. So why are we so hung up on how much we weigh? A lot of our orientation to weight has to do with that height/weight chart that used to be a fixture in our doctor's office. The chart said that if you are this old and this tall you should weigh this much. In truth, not many of us weighed what that chart said we should. How could it? We are all so different. We have different bone structures; we have different muscle structures. When was the last time you saw one of these charts? Most doctors threw them away years ago. They had no basis in reality. In truth, those charts were not an invention of the medical community at all; rather, the charts were produced by the insurance companies. The numbers on those charts represented an average of the heights and weights of the healthiest people, the people who were the least likely to be an insurance risk. In other words, if you fit within the parameters of the height/weight chart you were less likely to cost the insurance companies any money.

The first thing you have to do is change the way you think about the whole issue of weight. If you want to lose weight, you are missing the point. If you can come to the conclusion that you want to lose fat, you have a much clearer vision of the task at hand. You can then go about the business of eliminating fat from your body. Losing weight is a vague goal. Losing fat is much more specific. If you come to the conclusion that you want to lose fat rather than "weight," you can debunk about 75 percent of the myths that exist about "dieting."

Do you really care how much your insurance company thinks you should weigh? If you could meet that weight goal by cutting off your arm or your leg or both, would you do it? Do you want less muscle, or do you want less fat? Muscle weighs approximately two times more than fat. Ladies, if you were five pounds heavier on the scale but three dress sizes smaller, would you really care that you weighed more? Gentlemen, if you were five pounds heavier but were wearing pants with a waist size four inches smaller, would you care what your scale said? The point is that it is the fat that makes us uncomfortable with our appearance. When we look at ourselves in the mirror, it is the fat that we would like to eliminate. Your weight isn't the problem. Fat is the real enemy.

HOW DO I MEASURE FAT LOSS?

If you want to lose fat, you will need to find a way to see if your situation is improving. Again, the scale gives us only a partial look at what is happening to our bodies. If you could look at your total weight on the scale, and separate water, muscle, bone, hair, and nails from the weight of fat, then you would really have a tool to monitor your progress. Such a method of measurement exists. It is called a body-fat percentage measurement. There are many ways to measure the amount of fat on your body. Some are expensive, some are inexpensive. Some are accurate, some are not. The cheapest way to measure your body fat is just to notice how your clothes fit. Do they fit better? Are you wearing your "skinny pants"? Do your clothes no longer fit at all? The most cost-effective way to measure your body fat is to use a device called a skin fold caliper. The skin fold caliper can range in price from $5 at your local drugstore to $1,000 from a medical supplier, or you can have a professional take this measurement for $15 to $30. This device works by pinching the skin in several specific areas of your body and measuring the size of what you've pinched with the calipers. The manufacturer provides a formula for those measurements so you can determine your body-fat percentage. The more expensive the skin fold caliper, the more accurate, but even the least expensive gives you a fairly decent progress report. All calipers, regardless of price, come with directions. Each manufacturer recommends a different formula, and all you have to do is fill in the blanks and do the multiplication. Then there are high-tech, high-cost methods. Some weigh you in a tank of water, some use X rays (these are mostly found in scientific or academic settings, and if you had access to them you could expect to pay $500 or more). No matter which body-fat measurement you choose, your weight on the scale is only a part of the mathematical formula. Your weight on the scale is also only a part of your final reading.

When you get a body-fat measurement, you are usually given three numbers: your total weight on the scale, the percentage of your total weight that is comprised of lean muscle, bone, hair, nails, and water, and the percentage of your total weight that is made up of fat. For example, if you weigh 200 pounds and have a body-fat percentage of 25 percent, that really means that you have 150 pounds of water, muscle, organs, hair, and nails and 50 pounds of fat. This doesn't mean that you need to lose 50 pounds In fact, you couldn't possibly lose 50 pounds of fat. Fat serves many vital functions in your body, and you *need* some fat—not much, but some—to survive. Your body-fat percentage is simply a number you would like to reduce.

BODY-FAT GUIDELINES[3]	
MEN	**WOMEN**
< 10% Low body fat	< 15% Low body fat
10–20% Optimal range	15–25% Optimal range
21–25% Moderately high	26–30% Moderately high
> 31% Very high	> 35% Very high

Source: Power and Dodd

By now the goal is clear. Fat loss is the goal. Fat is what you want less of. If you reduce the amount of fat on your body, you will look better. If you reduce the amount of fat on your body, you will fit into the clothes you want to wear. If you reduce the amount of fat on your body, you will feel sexier and more appealing. If you reduce the amount of fat on your body, you will alleviate, if not solve, all of those vanity issues. However, you are still missing the point of it all. The point is that not only will you look better, but you will feel better. Feeling better really means improving your health. With the exception of not smoking, reducing fat and becoming more active are the greatest preventive measures there are, and doing them will greatly reduce your chances of serious health problems and many also increase your longevity.

It is estimated that over 50 percent of our nation's population is overweight, and that more than 30 million Americans suffer from obesity. There are more people on a diet today than there were last year, more people eating fat-free foods, and more people exercising than at any other time in history, and yet there are more people who are overweight. What was once considered a vanity issue has mushroomed into a problem so vast it is now a national health crisis.

The governmental agency devoted to help solve this problem of obesity is none other than the Centers for Disease Control. Traditionally when we think of this agency, we think of vaccinations for the most horrific diseases like smallpox or polio, monitoring Ebola breakouts, hepatitis contagion, or even the spread of AIDS. Few people know that obesity and inactivity are linked to the number one cause of death for American adults. Improper nutrition, inactivity, overweight, and obesity have been inextricably linked to heart attack and other cardiopulmonary maladies, respiratory ailments, atherosclerosis and circulatory illnesses, brain illnesses such as Alzheimer's disease, and many cancers. Aside from quitting tobacco use, reducing the amount of fat on your body and becoming more active are the surest and most proven methods for disease prevention.

YOUR BODY BILL

The real problem with "dieting" is that the mind-set is too temporary. When we think of going on a diet it is just for a few days, or a few weeks, or a couple of months. Unfortunately, we only enjoy the results of "dieting" for a short period of time and then we're "dieting" again. Let's change the whole notion around. Let's change the goals. Make this a lifelong change. Why don't we make the real goal a long-term goal? Why don't you make up your mind here and now that the real goal is to live to be 100 years old?

For each decade that you live, life hands you a bill. You started smoking in high school? Life will eventually hand you a bill. You drank too much, partied too much, stayed up too late in your twenties? Life hands you a bill. You worked too hard, kept strange hours, and had too much stress in your thirties? Life will hand you a bill in your forties. You never exercised, ate the wrong foods, and didn't attend to your health in your forties? Life will hand you a bill in your fifties. You burned the candle at both ends, you toiled so the kids got through college, you toiled so there would be enough in the 401(k), you stressed and fretted and worried so much that you forgot to enjoy a minute of your fifties? Life will hand you a bill in your sixties. Became completely inactive in your seventies? Life will make you pay that bill in your eighties.

It doesn't have to be that way! At the age of 50, George Foreman became the heavyweight champion of the world. At age 64, Dr. Sherman Bull made it to the summit of Mt. Everest. Jack LaLanne celebrated his seventieth birthday by swimming across San Francisco Bay, towing a rowboat with his wife and children in it! These weren't just publicity stunts; they did these amazing things to prove that they could be done. The point is that with all the breakthroughs in medical science, there is no reason at all why most of us cannot meet the goal of celebrating our hundredth birthday. Look at the statistics. In 1960, there were about 3,000 people in the world who were 100 years old. In 1995, there were more than 54,000. It is expected that there will be more than 2,700,000 centenarians in the year 2050.[4] Right here, right now, decide what your body bill is going to look like in ten years. You can change it. You can use The Equation and turn the numbers in your body bill upside down.

LOOK AT THE PROBLEM IN REVERSE

Changing your life takes a vision and a visionary approach to turn things around. It has been said that a visionary sees the end result and works the problem backward to right here, right now. See the results you want to get, see yourself in your golden years, see the possibilities of a rich full life, a life with quality, a life with vitality. Now work your way backward to today and you will discover your game plan or strategy. The game plan is what you can do today, tomorrow, next month, next year, and ten years from now. The important part is today—what can you do right now?

You want to get rid of some fat? Look at the problem in reverse. You didn't put this weight on last night while you were sleeping; it happened over a period of time. You may look quite different than you did a few years ago. You may be heavier today than the day you graduated from high school or college. If, after the age of 20, you gained two pounds every year, you would be 40 pounds heavier at the age of 40. This syndrome is called creeping obesity. In fact, creeping obesity is occurring for most of us, and it is a very subtle process. We become less active as we get older, we have less time to spend on ourselves when we take our first job, and less time when we get married, and even less time when we have children. Our responsibilities prevent us from exercising as much as we would like, and our hectic schedules prevent us from eating as well as we should. The changes in your lifestyle caused you to be heavier than you would like to be! If you can adjust your lifestyle, even slightly, to do more of the activities you are already doing and eating in a more conscious manner, you can completely reverse the syndrome of weight gain.

SMALL, SLOW, AND SURE

You cannot rid yourself of all the fat and weight today. The problem with most "diets," the real reason why they don't work, is that the goal is to lose "weight" and to lose it quickly. The unspoken fault with this philosophy is that you are eating and/or exercising in a way that you will not be able to sustain in the long run. At some point you will ease up, or go back to what you were doing before, and sooner or later you end up in the same place. Even if you had liposuction performed so that you did lose all that fat today, if you did not change the way you were eating and/or exercising, you would continue to gain fat.

Certain celebrities are a perfect example of this. They need to lose 35 pounds in three months. They do exactly what most commercial diets suggest: They go on a severely restricted diet. They exercise for hours each and every day. They reach their goal. Weeks after they finish filming that project they go back to eating normally, and in no time at all they are back where they started. Most people have seen the television show *Survivor*. The contestants are in a remote location for more than a month. They are basically starving. They lose a tremendous amount of weight in a very short time. In a matter of months after they return home, they are heavier than when they reached the island.

The more extreme your departure from what you are currently doing, the greater your chances for failure. However, if you give yourself the luxury of time, you can take a less radical approach. The smaller the change, the greater the possibility that you can sustain that change for the rest of your life. Because you want to enjoy the results you get for the rest of your life, the goal is to change your lifestyle, not to be on a diet.

The only answer is to do something with the intention of doing it for the rest of your life. With most diets, if you cheat for a meal, or go off the diet for a week, you have blown it. By using The Equation, you will have many opportunities to get back on track after any such detour. Once you begin, you can always work The Equation. With The Equation, you are always on the right road. If you happen to get off the road, your journey isn't over, and you can easily get back on track.

THE TRANSITION FROM CONTEMPLATION TO ACTION

Beginning to use The Equation is effortless. Much like dipping your toes in the water to check the temperature, you can make the transition from thinking about what you want to do and in small stages start to do something to change your situation. Again, the suggestion is to change one simple thing and continue to do it for the rest of your life. Much of your success with The Equation will come from altering your behavior ever so slightly. These small habitual changes can and will eventually lead to amazing results over the long term.

As we stated earlier, The Equation represents everything we know to be true about diet and exercise. We have narrowed down all of your options to only those that have been scientifically proven to work. Your own experimentation is limited to what works for you within these guidelines.

Here is an example of what could be your first experiment. We all have a different response to the foods we eat. For some, eating foods with a high sugar content causes them to have sugar cravings throughout the day. For others, having a protein-rich first meal provides greater energy throughout the day. All of us, whether through habit or preference, usually start our days in a similar fashion. Over the next week, expand your horizons and try a different breakfast each day. The experiment is to learn which foods work best for you and which are most beneficial for the purposes of realizing your dreams of physical transformation. Next week, eat a breakfast containing only one of the following foods: fruit, cereal, or eggs. As part of your experiment, note any cravings you have through the day. Note how much energy you have. Note how long it takes for you to be ready for your next meal. Note how frequently you need snacks with each of these different breakfasts.

By the end of the week, you should know in no uncertain terms what type of breakfast meal best serves you. You will know that if you eat a certain food, you will get a certain response. In general terms, you will have more energy and "feel" better just by eating this particular food. More often than not, this type of breakfast will also serve your purposes for either maintaining your weight or allowing you to reduce your weight. When you do not eat what is best for you, you feel sluggish and less efficient. As a result, you may make a habit of eating the same general foods for this first meal. When you can determine what works best for you and then incorporate that into habitual behavior, not only can you achieve results but you also can continue to enjoy those results for the rest of your life.

PART TWO

EQUATION

for a

LEAN LIFESTYLE

As a scientist you are creating an experiment. You are also the subject of your own experiment, so a certain amount of care must be taken to ensure your safety. Almost as important, you want to conduct your experiment with enough attention so that you can determine if what you are trying worked, and if it worked, why it worked.

The scientist first begins with a control, a baseline that will provide proof of any changes. Your baseline is a careful assessment of where you are at this very moment and where you would like to go. You have lived inside of your body for quite a while, and you are an absolute expert on the subject. Note how you feel. Ponder any health problems you have had, and also consider how often you are sick or how susceptible you are to colds and flu. Take an honest look at your energy level. Is it as high as that of others around you? Do you like to be outdoors, or do you prefer being indoors? Are you on the go, constantly moving and doing, or do you prefer to be sitting, resting, or watching television? If you prefer more sedentary activities, what effect does this have on your life? Are you less active than you would like to be? Has this had a negative effect on your social life? Has your energy level had any negative effects on your work life or career? On a scale of 1 to 10, how would you rate your energy level? What about your energy level would you like to change? On a scale of 1 to 10, where would you like your energy level to be? Step onto the scale and take careful notes about your weight and size. Is this a "normal" weight for you? Is your weight a little high, or is this the highest it has ever been? How do your clothes fit? Do you have several sections in your closet devoted to different sizes of slacks? Are you wearing your "fat pants" or your "skinny pants"? Compared to the past, how large is your waist? Your hips? Your thighs? The underside of your arms? Your buttocks? Are there particular areas of your body you would desperately like to change? How do you feel at the beach? How do you feel in intimate situations? The more detailed you can be when answering questions such as these, the more easily you can determine when change is occurring.

We can assure you that you will experience a change. However, change, especially the change of losing fat, can be difficult. First, the human body is not really equipped to rid itself of fat easily. Human beings are still on the planet because we have an intensely heightened and perfected survival mechanism. Over the thousands of years that we have been around, a large part of survival has meant living through periods when there was not enough fresh water to drink and/or not enough food to eat. Our bodies are equipped with innate devices that will see us through times of need and times of uncertainty. Our greatest defense against starvation is the fat on our bodies. Our fat is a vast storage depot for the fuel we need to keep our motor running. We require a certain amount of energy just to stay alive. It takes energy to keep our hearts beating, our blood pumping, and our lungs breathing. That energy comes from the food we eat. When there is no food, our survival mechanism is called to work, and our fat cells release energy from our storage depot so we may continue to live.

To call upon these fat reserves takes a proven strategy. We have much information on this subject, and the best of that information reveals that you will have the most success not by shocking your system but by making slow, small, and gradual changes that allow your survival mechanisms to relax. In other words, if you go on a highly restrictive diet, you shock your body. This shock puts all of your food-related survival mechanisms on alert. In the end, your restrictive diet will deliver the exact opposite results from the ones you desire. On the highly restrictive diet you may indeed lose a little weight, but as soon as you return to eating normally, you will gain back all the weight that you lost plus a little bit more, ending up with a greater percentage of fat than you had before you began the original diet. However, when these survival mechanisms are allowed to relax, your body feels comfortable and confident releasing fat from its storage depot. In essence, you could make one tiny change for the rest of your life and have far greater results than if you "dieted" for the rest of your life. It takes some time for your natural survival instincts to relax, and keeping them relaxed takes a little maintenance, but if you can be consistent, you will create the foundation for lasting change.

Anyone can lose a few pounds. ***Lasting change is the goal***. These small changes you will make to your everyday routine are completely painless and require very little effort. When you can make one small and painless adjustment to your routine and make that adjustment part of your new routine, you have created a *new* habit. If you can allow that habit to become a consistent pattern of behavior for a certain duration of time, you have successfully made an adjustment to your lifestyle.

The key issues that all dieters face are completely ignored by commercial diets. In reality, you have gained the weight you now want to lose by altering your lifestyle and your behavior to promote weight gain. There are many patterns of behavior that most lean people have, and these are patterns of behavior that you must learn or relearn. We have labeled these habits the cornerstones of a lean lifestyle. Throughout this section of the book, you will be encouraged to emulate the lean lifestyle. These cornerstones will serve as a foundation for your transformation, and once in place, will enable you to maintain the results you achieve for the remainder of your life. Over the next three weeks you will make some very small adjustments to your life: learning to properly hydrate your body, eating several small meals throughout the day, becoming consistent with the times you eat, and creating the perfect size for each meal. Soon these small adjustments will become new habits. By being consistent and vigilant, these habits will blossom into a new lifestyle. In a few months, you will look in the mirror and realize that your new lifestyle created a new you.

Losing weight is much like being a safecracker. All that separates you from the treasure waiting behind the locked door is the right combination. At this moment you are not certain which number could open that lock, but over the next three weeks you will discover the combination. During your first week, you will develop a new habit, which can be seen as one element of the combination. If that does not open the lock to the treasure, you add another element. If that does not open the lock, you add yet another element to that combination. If, after the next three weeks, you have not reached the treasure, there are still more layers to be revealed, but you will have developed the cornerstones of a lean mentality. With these cornerstones, this foundation, this new lifestyle in place, you can achieve any goal you set. Without this foundation, without a new lifestyle in place, you will never be able to make the changes you desire.

CHAPTER THREE

STEP ONE

Equation for Water–Drinking Your Fat Away

Over the next week, you will make one minor adjustment to your daily routine. It is your goal to turn this minor adjustment into a habit—something you do each and every day—and continue practicing this habit until the habit becomes part of your lifestyle. The goal is to create a new lifestyle, a lean lifestyle. Over time this new lifestyle will help to create a new you.

There has been much research and study on breaking habits, or in this case, creating new habits. Much of this research has been done by behavioral scientists and also perfected by alcohol and drug cessation centers, or twelve-step programs. Starting with Alcoholics Anonymous, and continuing with the hundreds of drug treatment centers around the world, the notion of breaking a habit—or even an addiction—has been refined into science. What we know from their painstaking decades of trial and error is that it takes repetition and time to break or create a habit. Once the habit has been broken or created, it can take 12 to 18 months for that habit to really become a part of your lifestyle.

Your goal is to create a new habit and allow that new habit to become part of your new lifestyle, a component of the new you. During this first week, you will begin the process of creating a new habit. You will need to be consistent with this adjustment for at least 21 days to create a new habit, and be consistent in that habit to become part of your new lifestyle. Again, these minor adjustments are painless and effortless. They require little or no sacrifice and only a small amount of attention to complete the task. However, these adjustments, although minor, can have dramatic, even miraculous results over the course of your lifetime. These small changes will have a greater effect than any "diet." These small changes are the foundation on which a new you can be built.

The first small adjustment you will make is the most basic. The first step in the equation concerns the most essential, the most basic substance on the planet—water. Water is the source of all life on Earth and covers more than two-thirds of its surface. Overwhelmingly, your body is comprised of water. You could go without eating for weeks and months, but only a day or two without water. Other than air and the ability to breathe, water is the most essential element to sustaining life. Water also represents the safest, simplest, and most effective method to eliminate body fat.

Although drinking water does not burn off fat in and of itself, the physiological process that occurs with water consumption is simple to comprehend. The first and most important aspect to drinking more water is that you will feel less hungry, and feel satisfied even when you eat less.

One of the great lessons of creating a lean lifestyle is understanding the distinction between comfortably full or "satisfied" and full or "uncomfortably stuffed." By increasing your intake of water, your stomach is never allowed to feel empty. Consequently, when you eat, you will not have to eat as much to reach a level where you are no longer hungry. If you are still unsatisfied after eating, you can drink additional water until you do feel comfortably full or "satisfied." When you learn to eat only to the level where you are no longer hungry, you have done much to create a lean lifestyle, and water is the key to feeling satisfied throughout the day.

The importance of properly hydrating your body cannot and should not be overlooked. Hydration, better known as having enough water in your body, is a key to making your body operate efficiently. If you were a car, we could safely say that food is very much like putting gas in the tank. Drinking enough water is very much like having oil in your car. You need to keep the oil at a certain level for the car to run efficiently. The oil in your car keeps all the different parts lubricated and moving. Everything inside your car is completely dependent on oil to work and work properly. If you did not have oil in your car, the engine would "freeze," and no moving part in your car would ever move again. Essentially the car would be dead. The same is true for you. Water affects your energy level, the way you feel, the way your organs function, the way you move, how much you eat, the way you digest your food, and how much of that food is used.

Many of us do not take in enough water to keep our bodies working at the highest possible level. How are you feeling right now? Is your energy level as high as it could be? Increasing your water intake can have dramatic and immediate results. Don't take our word for it—try it yourself. Before you read any farther, drink a tall glass of water, refill the glass, and then come back to read on. Most of us are looking for the quick fix when we consider dieting. We all want results and we want them now. It is hard to imagine, but drinking enough water can actually offer you the quickest result. Inside our bodies, we are a vast roadway of veins and arteries. Nutrients are carried over these roads (our bloodstream) to the various parts of our body. When we are dehydrated, the volume of blood decreases sharply. As a result, our veins and arteries experience something that would look like a traffic jam. The blood, or cars, is still moving, but not as quickly as everyone on the road would like. As a result, commuters are late in arriving at their destinations. When we are properly hydrated, traffic moves smoothly and much more quickly. In other words, when you are properly hydrated, there is an increase in plasma levels, and nutrients are better able to travel to the place where they are needed, and as a result, you notice a dramatic difference in your energy level. Just to illustrate the point, drink that second glass of water. Now fill up a third glass and sip it as you read the next several paragraphs.

It may seem simple, so simple that it verges on stupidity. But invariably people forget how important water is. When Dan is on the set with a celebrity, he is always at the ready with a bottle of water. When an actor is doing a particularly emotional or physically demanding scene, he always makes certain that he or she is drinking water between takes. When his or her energy is lagging, Dan offers a bottle. (Keep sipping that water so you can see for yourself.)

It is easy to tell someone to drink more water. In fact, you have probably heard it before. But you really need to experience what proper hydration can mean to you. Over the next week, you are going to begin the process of becoming conscious about drinking water. Once you have started creating the new habit of hydrating yourself to proper levels, you will be hooked. It will do much more for you than just help you reduce your weight. It will aid your body in every way. This is a habit that you definitely need to incorporate into your lifestyle. (Keep sipping!)

An accountant friend of ours has had a bad back for years. He saw doctor after doctor. He had X rays and MRIs. He took pain medication and muscle relaxants. He saw chiropractors and massage therapists. But he couldn't get relief from the pain. After tax season, he went on vacation. After the first three days his back froze up and he spent the rest of vacation holed up in his hotel room, unable to enjoy himself or to relax. He returned home, and things improved to the point that he could at least move. He consulted with a personal trainer, thinking that specific exercises might be able to help. The first thing the trainer asked was, "How much water do you drink?" Like most of us, his answer was, "Not much." The trainer continued his inquiry. "When you were on vacation, how much water were you drinking?" The man replied, "None. I was just sitting around the pool drinking beer. I was trying to relax." The trainer asked one final question. "How much water did you drink today?" The man answered, "Well, none. I had some coffee this morning, but no plain water." The trainer explained that alcohol and caffeine are chemicals that significantly dehydrate the human body. The fact that the man was not drinking any water at all made dehydration even more severe. The trainer felt that exercise would help his bad back, but told him that more than anything else, water would be the solution. The trainer put the man on the same hydration plan you are just beginning. After just the first day, his back pain diminished considerably. After the first week, the pain was completely gone. At this point he returned to his doctor's office and reported his experience. His doctor agreed that it could've just been a matter of proper hydration. The man asked, "Why didn't anyone tell me that?" Apologetically, the doctor said that it didn't even occur to him to pass on that information—the solution to the problem was so simple that it had completely escaped him. As a token of his sorrow, the doctor retook the MRI images at his own expense. To their surprise, the difference between the "before" and "after" images was dramatic. Before the accountant began this hydration plan, the disks on his spine appeared to be black spots between the vertebrae. After he began regularly and properly hydrating himself, his disks appeared to be white and plump on the MRI images. The accountant has continued this hydration program and has been without any back pain ever since that time.

The moral of the story is that when you are properly hydrated, everything—all of your bodily functions—works better. As more water flushes through the digestive tract, more and more harmful toxins are purged from your system. Within the first week, you will notice that your body seems to be working better. In this first week, you may experience an improvement in your clarity of thought. As water is the best conductor of electricity, the neurons firing in the brain reach their intended destination quicker and more effectively. In the second week, you might notice improvements in your skin and hair quality as harmful toxins are flushed out of your system. In the third week, you will experience an overall feeling of wellness. You will feel more alert, you may eliminate chronic headaches or chronic fatigue, you will become more attentive and more energized, and you'll experience the benefits of your bodily systems operating at full capacity.

By now you have finished your third glass of water. If not, finish the rest of the glass. Close your eyes, take a few deep breaths, and make some notes about the way you feel. Do you have more energy than when you began reading this chapter? Are you more focused? The process of hydrating your body is remarkable. With proper hydration there is an almost immediate reversal of fatigue. You should be experiencing a similar feeling at this very moment. By increasing your intake of water, you have increased the volume of blood in your system, and nutrients can be delivered to where they are needed most. If you were engaged in strenuous activity, those nutrients would be delivered to whichever muscles were at work. Because you are presently engaged in a mental activity, those nutrients are being delivered to your brain, and as a result you feel more focused. That is what is meant by an immediate result. We must warn you that with this increase in water you will be in the bathroom more frequently. We suggest that you stop drinking about three hours prior to bedtime, or you may wake up frequently and disrupt your normal sleeping patterns.

Water, and the process of hydrating, will also give you a relatively quick result in terms of weight loss. Over the course of this next week you will learn a great lesson about the human body. The human body conserves all it can. Human beings have an amazing built-in survival mechanism, and over the next week you will be keenly aware of how you can coax your body into feeling comfortable enough to let go of what it would normally hold in reserve.

During the course of a normal day you excrete about 1.5 liters of water each day. Because such a great percentage of your body is made up of water, it is essential that you replenish that amount of water plus a little bit more. We recommend that you drink *at least* 2 liters or about 64 ounces of water per day. If you do not drink that much water, your body is unsure if it will ever drink again. Consequently, your body holds on to as much water as it can. Typically we call this "retaining water," but it really is just our bodies trying to protect us. Our genetic code doesn't realize that we are living in the twenty-first century. It doesn't realize there is such a thing as a water tap. It is just doing its job. If you go without water for more than 48 hours, you are in grave danger. Your body is merely trying to save your life.

SIGNS AND SYMPTOMS OF LOW LEVELS OF HYDRATION

Chronic constipation and headaches

Dry mouth, skin, and nasal membranes

Increased heart rate

Increased blood pressure

Water retention

Muscle constriction

Again, the goal is to take in enough water, make hydrating your body a habit, and make that habit a component of a lean lifestyle that helps to create a new you. The first step in that process is to allow your body to feel comfortable. On the first day you may not find enough time to drink all that water. The second day will get a little easier. In these first two days you will certainly notice that you never feel truly hungry, and you will probably also note a dramatic improvement in your energy level. On the third day you will urinate more frequently, and this pattern of drinking and relieving yourself will become more regular. You may notice that your joints move more easily or that you are more flexible. You may notice a change in the way you are digesting your food. At the end of week two, you may notice improvements to the quality of your skin and hair. At the end of the third week, the time when proper hydration becomes a habit, you notice that something is different when you look in the mirror. At the end of this three-week period, from just the process of properly hydrating your body, you may experience weight loss because of a reduction in the amount of food you are eating. In learning to strike a balance in your level of hunger and eating only until you feel comfortably full, you will experience a loss of fat and weight. For some, this small change will provide all the results they are looking for.

THE PROGRAM

Drink 64 ounces of water throughout the day.

WORKING THE EQUATION

Remember, water is absorbed better when it's cool. It absorbs better when sipped. When gulped, the body tends to excrete rather than absorb.

Fresh-squeezed lemon or lime can add some zip to plain water.

Drinking before and/or after meals may help you feel a bit fuller and reduce the quantity of food you are likely to eat.

Use a bicycle water bottle for your daily water supply; refill it as you drink it up.

Avoid or limit caffeinated drinks like coffee, tea, or soda. Caffeine causes the body to excrete water and become dehydrated.

Modify

- Drink a glass of water before every meal.
- Fruit juice diluted with water is also a great way to make your own low-calorie drink.

Substitute

- Before going back for "seconds," have a glass of water and wait 10 minutes.
- Drink decaffeinated tea and coffee. Try substituting green tea for your morning coffee.
- If you are a coffee drinker, have a glass of water before each cup of coffee.

Shift

- Use decaffeinated drinks.
- Make drinking water a healthy habit, or a new job you want to complete every day like brushing your teeth. Drink 8 glasses of water a day or take a water bottle and refill it throughout the day or buy a case of water bottles and finish four 16-ounce bottles each day.

WHAT TO EXPECT THIS WEEK

Just by drinking 64 ounces of water each day, you will notice that you are operating more efficiently. You will feel an increase in energy and clarity of thought, and possibly an improvement in your digestion. By drinking more fluids, most people will naturally eat smaller amounts of food. Again, the most important lesson is to learn to accept feeling comfortably full or satisfied, and not to eat until you feel "full." During this week you may find that striking this balance between "satisfied" and "full" will not only have a positive effect on your waistline, but may also allow you to feel more energized, alert, and more effective. Over the course of this week, you should become 1 or 2 pounds lighter. By maintaining this level of hydration you may rid yourself of 4 to 6 pounds over the course of one year.

HOW TO USE THE BODY BILL

This week is crucial. Increasing your intake of water is essential for a lean lifestyle and also as a building block for your physical transformation. It is important to begin tracking what you are doing to create this change. It has been proven that just using a journal for notations such as these can aid in the process of weight loss. It will become increasingly more important to use the body bill provided, and it is strongly recommended that you get in the habit of using the pages provided.

On each body bill you will see the hours of the day marked 1 to 16. Hour 1 is the moment you wake up. Every two hours you will drink 16 ounces of water. When you have completed that task, simply make a check mark in the space provided. It is that easy.

BODY BILL

DAY 1

Hour	Water	Completed
1		
	16 ounces WATER	_____
2		
3		
4		
	16 ounces WATER	_____
5		
6		
7	16 ounces WATER	_____
8		
9		
	16 ounces WATER	_____
10		
11		
12		
13		
14		
15		
16		

Difficulties and Insights

_____

_____

_____

_____

_____

_____

BODY BILL

DAY 2

Hour	Water		Completed
1			
2	16 ounces WATER		_____
3			
4			
5	16 ounces WATER		_____
6			
7	16 ounces WATER		_____
8			
9			
10	16 ounces WATER		_____
11			
12			
13			
14			
15			
16			

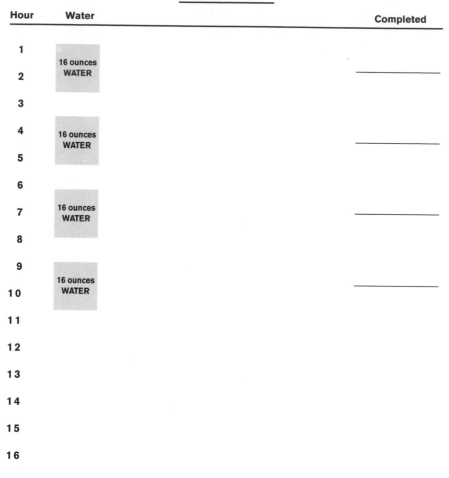

Difficulties and Insights

_____

_____

_____

_____

_____

_____

BODY BILL

DAY 3

Hour	Water		Completed
1			
	16 ounces WATER		_____
2			
3			
4	16 ounces WATER		_____
5			
6			
7	16 ounces WATER		_____
8			
9			
	16 ounces WATER		_____
10			
11			
12			
13			
14			
15			
16			

Difficulties and Insights

_____

_____

_____

_____

_____

_____

BODY BILL

DAY 4

Hour	Water		Completed
1			
2	16 ounces WATER		_____
3			
4	16 ounces WATER		
5			_____
6			
7	16 ounces WATER		_____
8			
9			
10	16 ounces WATER		_____
11			
12			
13			
14			
15			
16			

Difficulties and Insights

_____

_____

_____

_____

_____

_____

BODY BILL

DAY 5

Hour	Water		Completed
1			
2	16 ounces WATER		_____
3			
4	16 ounces WATER		_____
5			
6			
7	16 ounces WATER		_____
8			
9	16 ounces WATER		_____
10			
11			
12			
13			
14			
15			
16			

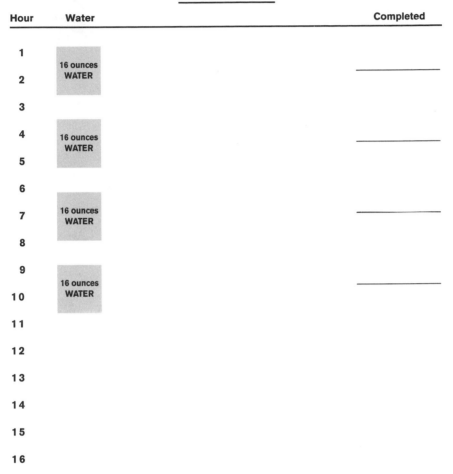

Difficulties and Insights

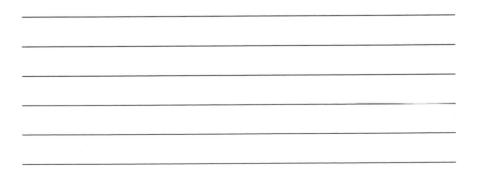

_____

_____

_____

_____

_____

_____

BODY BILL

DAY 6

Hour	Water		Completed
1			
2	16 ounces WATER		———————
3			
4	16 ounces WATER		———————
5			
6			
7	16 ounces WATER		———————
8			
9			
10	16 ounces WATER		———————
11			
12			
13			
14			
15			
16			

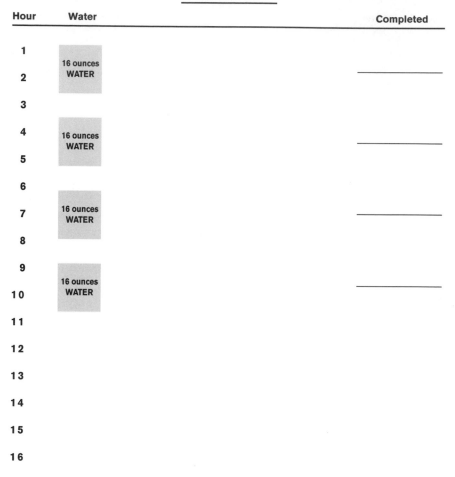

Difficulties and Insights

_____

_____

_____

_____

_____

_____

BODY BILL

DAY 7

Hour	Water		Completed
1			
	16 ounces WATER		_____
2			
3			
4			
	16 ounces WATER		_____
5			
6			
7	16 ounces WATER		_____
8			
9			
	16 ounces WATER		_____
10			
11			
12			
13			
14			
15			
16			

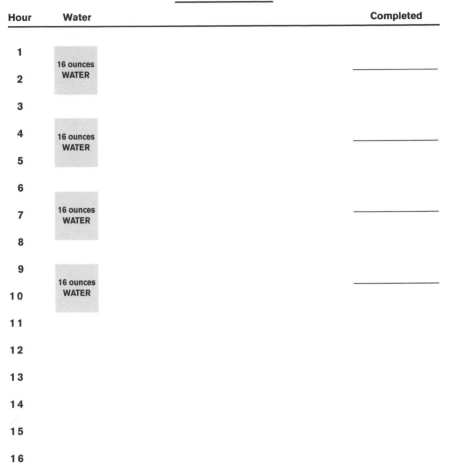

Difficulties and Insights

_____

_____

_____

_____

_____

CHAPTER FOUR

STEP TWO

Equation for Eating—
It's About Time

Like building a house, you are creating a foundation for a physical transformation—the new you. It is possible that by just drinking water and properly hydrating yourself, you solved your weight-loss dilemma. Over the next week, you will add another layer to your lifestyle, making only a slight adjustment to begin a new way of eating. Over the next week, you will become ultraconscious about when you eat, and even more consistent about what time you are eating.

There is a vast difference between the times when you *need* to eat and the times you *should* eat. Timing, as they say, is everything. Last week you learned a profound lesson. You now have a tangible understanding of how your body is equipped to survive, and if you can disarm your built-in survival mechanism, you can relax your body into releasing what it holds in storage. The human race has been able to survive hardship specifically because we have survival mechanisms. Aside from water, we also need food, and the human body is equipped with a very sophisticated starvation protection device. The primary tool for that device is the fat we have on our bodies. This starvation-protection device is tremendously sensitive, and the reason why most diets do not work is that your intake of food becomes so low that your starvation-protection device becomes activated. When that device is activated, it stores almost all the food you eat as fat and burns off only the bare minimum. Your task this week is to learn how to disarm your own starvation-protection device. Just like you did by hydrating your body in week one, you can and will coax your body into releasing what has been stored into your fat cells, but again, this is a process. You cannot and should not expect your body to release all of your stored fat in just one week! This week you are taking the first step in that process. An important component of your new lifestyle is making a simple adjustment to the way you eat, so you do not store away any additional fat. While you cannot eliminate all of your fat in one week, you can begin to lay the groundwork for that to occur.

The difference between when you *need to* eat and when you *should* eat is subtle, but it can be the difference between failure and success, between being lean and being overweight. By the time you feel that you need to eat, chances are you have waited too long. By the time you begin to feel really hungry, you will usually eat too much food too quickly. When this occurs, your body will be forced to store more of the food you eat within your fat cells.

This week you will actually short-circuit this process by scheduling your meals. This week, it is essential that you try to eat at exactly the same times each day. Eating at the same times each day will get your body into a rhythm, a routine. Your body will quickly adapt to this routine and will begin to rely on the fact that it will be fed. After about five days, your body will begin to understand that it is being taken care of and it does not have to be on alert to prevent starvation. As this mechanism begins to relax its vigilance, you will begin to feel the difference in the way your body is processing the food you eat. By eating at roughly the same times each and every day, not only will you have a tendency to not put on any additional fat, but your body will naturally begin the process of burning off stored fat.

The word *metabolism* is used and misused frequently. Many are concerned that their metabolism is "too slow." For most, not eating frequently enough, going for long or extended periods of time between meals, and eating too much at one sitting all play a role in this phenomenon. What is really at issue is the way the human body is wired to combat starvation. In part, eating at specific times will solve many issues pertaining to the starvation-protection mechanism. However, you must also eat frequently to prevent the starvation-protection device from being activated. It is most advantageous to eat several smaller meals throughout the day, and it is recommended that you eat at least five meals per day. This week, you should eat what you would normally eat during the course of the day, but spread that food out over these many meals. In other words, you are eating a smaller breakfast, lunch, and dinner, and having a snack between meals. Your meals will be separated by about 2½ to 3 hours to assure that your food has been digested. As you create an eating schedule, and eat these five meals at the same times each day, your starvation-protection device will be disarmed. Consequently, this effectively speeds your metabolism, as your body will use up most of the food you eat for fuel and store less of it for later use.

Eating several meals throughout the day and at the same time may at first seem a little regimented, but strangely enough, you will actually develop a sense of freedom. In reality, you have no choice—you must eat to survive. By eating at regular times you are creating a routine, a new pattern of behavior, a new habit, and eventually a new lifestyle. By designating specific feeding times, you eliminate the choice of eating or not eating. Remember, you must eat in order to live. The only thing you are eliminating now is thinking about when you eat. When it is time to eat, you may eat any kind of food you choose. By eliminating the choice of when you eat, you can be fairly certain that you will have successfully short-circuited your starvation-protection device.

NATURAL NUTRITION

The intention of this book is to suggest lifestyle patterns that aid the process of eliminating body fat naturally. Regarding when you eat, many examples in nature are relevant. The notion of natural nutrition is not a recommendation for living off of insects and tree bark; rather, it is a suggested lifestyle shift that is more in keeping with our true nature.

There are many examples of how the typical twenty-first-century lifestyle that most of us lead has caused us to become less lean than we would like to be. Our world is so different from that of our great-grandparents, our grandparents, and even our parents. Since the Industrial Revolution, more and more of the world's population has moved into urban centers. In the last hundred years, most Americans have shifted from an agrarian society to that of urban workers with a nine-to-five workday, putting in forty hours per week on the job. In the last ten years, most of us have found ourselves working even longer hours, more homes have two working parents, and we have less time to spend with our families and loved ones— and much less time to spend on ourselves. These shifts have led to innumerable lifestyle changes that have dramatically affected our lives, our relationships, and even the amount of fat we carry around with us.

The most harmful effects of urbanization center on our detachment from the earth. When people lived off of the land and were more in tune with nature and their surroundings, they also tended to carry less fat. When we grew our own crops and raised our own animals for food, we appreciated what we put into our bodies much more than we do today. By just spending the energy to grow this food or catch it, we were much more appreciative of having it.

In our society, the most abundant on earth, the most bountiful in the history of the planet, most of us live in city centers and are quite removed from the process of harvesting, picking, killing, and catching. For most of us, meat does not come from a four-legged animal, meat is wrapped in Styrofoam and plastic, and we find it in our local grocery store right next to the poultry and fish. Bread does not come from wheat fields; rice doesn't come from paddies; they both come in plastic bags. Fruits and vegetables are both on the same aisle. Our detachment from the whole process is so extreme that we don't even have to get out of our cars to hunt and gather. When we grew our own crops and raised or caught our own meats, our food was fresh, we wasted less of it, and we were much more in touch with the natural order of our world.

There are many things that we can do to create a more natural approach to living and consequently a natural approach to ridding ourselves of fat. Nature offers us many examples that are worthy of emulation. If you have ever woken up before sunrise, you know firsthand that birds and other creatures are already well into their day and going about the work of finding their first meal, and they eat several meals throughout the day. As night approaches these creatures are settling in for the evening and for the most part are finished with their day as the sun sets. This type of daily clock serves as the best schedule for most of us. To create a greater sense of balance in your daily schedule and your eating patterns, it may be advantageous for you to follow a more natural guideline. It is quite possible that this could be the missing link in your fat-loss program.

To keep yourself energized, it is essential that you eat frequently, and we suggest that you begin to eat several smaller meals throughout the day. Instead of the traditional three meals that most people eat, you will be much more successful in ridding yourself of fat if you eat at least five smaller meals per day. As you look at examples from nature, rarely do animals eat three square meals, nor do they continue to eat after they are satisfied. More typically, animals eat several meals during the day, and eat only until they are sated. Your first task is to begin eating your first meal within an hour after waking up, eat a small meal every 2½ to 3 hours, and finish your last meal at or shortly after sunset.

Without doubt, breakfast is the most important meal of the day. Many of us go without breakfast, and as a result we rob ourselves of the most fundamental process to set our metabolism at the highest possible speed, so that it quickly and efficiently processes the food we eat. After a full night of rest and many hours without food, the body needs to be nourished almost immediately. After all, you have not eaten for at least eight hours, so it stands to reason that you are hungry. If you can eat within an hour of waking, your body will respond almost immediately by becoming more alert and feeling energized. Much like clearing out the "cobwebs" after a full night's rest, all of your bodily functions are doing the same thing—waking up. As a result of the nutrients contained in your first meal, all of your bodily functions begin operating at their most efficient level. After waking, if you go more than one hour without this vital meal, you can set off the starvation-protection device and rob yourself of the opportunity to fuel the furnace of your metabolism to its highest possible setting.

When you eat within an hour of waking up, you set your metabolic rate to full speed ahead. After 2½ to 3 hours, your body has used up all of that food, and you need to replenish your fuel source. To continue to keep your metabolism on its highest setting, you need to eat at least four more meals. The last of these meals should be eaten at or shortly after sunset. After the sun sets, your body is naturally predisposed to wind down and rest. Physiologically, your temperature begins to drop, and vital functions like heartbeat and breathing begin to slow, until you are ready for sleep. These are your natural rhythms, and it is essential that your daily schedule reflect the example nature has set for you.

MAKING TIME

The largest obstacle you will face over the next week is time. You may have to bring your lunch to work with you, you may have to stock the refrigerator at the office, and you may have to force yourself to take breaks. All this takes time. We are all in a rush most of the time. Our hurriedness is definitely a major part of our weight problem. We are busier now than we have ever been. We spend less time on our family and friends, on hobbies and leisure, less time on vacation, less time reading, less time sleeping, and less time on ourselves than at any other point in the history of humankind. Today we are also fatter than we were last year, and we were fatter last year than we were the previous year. There are more people suffering from obesity than ever before. Time, or the lack of it, is not a small factor in this trend.

For those of you who (like us) are time-challenged, remind yourself of this fact: Your time is your own until you give it away. When attempting to reduce your body-fat percentage it is vital to take time for yourself when it comes to eating. To successfully absorb this notion of "making time," and incorporate it into your lifestyle, you must make the necessary preparation to ensure that you have food ready and available when you need it. Because most of us are on the go and "don't have time," when we finally get around to eating we are so hungry that we choose the quickest remedy, fast food. Fast food is at the root of our society's weight-loss dilemma. Fast-food franchises are everywhere you look and often are the only option when eating out. There is no surer way to increase the amount of fat on your body than to eat fast food. It becomes mandatory that you eliminate fast food from your diet, or at least reduce the number of times you eat fast food to the barest minimum.

The actual time you spend eating any given meal is equally important. If possible, it is best to eat your meals at a leisurely pace. Your mother and grandmother told you repeatedly, "Chew your food!" There are those of us who eat quickly and those who eat slowly, and it is important to note that a great many of the slow eaters are much leaner that the fast eaters. The digestive process is remarkable and can digest almost any nonmetallic object, but digestion can be aided a great deal when food particles are not so large. While you chew, a number of chemical reactions occur in the mouth, telling the digestive tract what is coming down the pipe and also releasing hormones into the bloodstream so that food can be digested. If you can chew each bite at least 20 times, your food will be digested easily and be burned more efficiently.

Eating at a leisurely pace also means that you are seated at a table without distraction from anything except good food or good company. When we eat on the run, at our desk at work, in the car while driving, or even while watching television, eating becomes an unconscious activity. It isn't that the food isn't as nourishing, but psychologically the fulfillment of that meal is not as great as it could be. An example of *conscious* eating is the family dinner. Not so long ago, the family ate its evening meal together each night at a designated time. Recent studies have shown that 90 percent of children who almost always eat a traditional dinner at home with other family members are not overweight and are much leaner than children who eat dinner without the family unit. The same studies indicate that this holds true for adults with or without children.[5] Making time to truly enjoy your food and the people who are important to you not only allows you to appreciate a meal but also provides an opportunity to form a stronger understanding and bond with those who are dear to you. Over the next week, make a habit of eating a traditional evening meal. Enjoy this meal and the company seated at the table. The sharing of meals, the "breaking of bread," is one of the most enjoyable events that can be shared. Making time for this traditional or shared meal can provide you with at least one hour of real quality time in your day.

THE PROGRAM

Look at what you typically eat during the course of an average day. Split that amount of food over five meals instead of one, two, or three meals. Eat what you would normally eat, just eat more frequently.

1. Begin your first meal within an hour after you wake up.
2. Eat a meal every 2½ to 3 hours.
3. Finish your fifth (and last) meal around sunset.
4. Eat these five meals at the same times each day for a week.

WORKING THE EQUATION

Preparation is key

You may have to stock the refrigerator at work, you may have to prepare food and take it with you, you may have to keep snacks in the car. You have a choice about *what* you eat, but you have no choice about *when* to eat.

Eat at a leisurely pace

By all means, enjoy your meal. Eat without the distractions of television, telephone, or newspapers or other reading materials. Avoid eating while driving or sitting at your desk. Take the time to enjoy your food.

Traditional meal

Have at least one meal per day seated at a table. Share this meal with friends, or family, or just make it special for yourself.

Chew your food well

Take your time. Get in the habit of chewing each bite twenty times, and not only will your digestive process work more efficiently, but you will also gain a greater satisfaction from eating and may even find yourself eating less.

WHAT TO EXPECT THIS WEEK

It is unreasonable to expect a tremendous result in terms of weight loss this week, but you may actually lose a pound or two. This is a process. What you are doing is gently coaxing your starvation-protection device into a state of relaxation. Over the next week, your body will begin to feel confident that it will be fed at regular intervals, and when this happens, your body can feel comfortable releasing energy stored within your body fat.

HOW TO USE THE BODY BILL

It has been proven that just using a journal to note your intake of food can aid in the process of weight loss. It will become more and more important to make notation of the foods you eat as you start the next chapters, so get in the habit now. For each day, simply make a check mark when you complete a meal and note what time you ate that meal. Be as consistent as you can with the timing of your meals.

BODY BILL

DAY 1

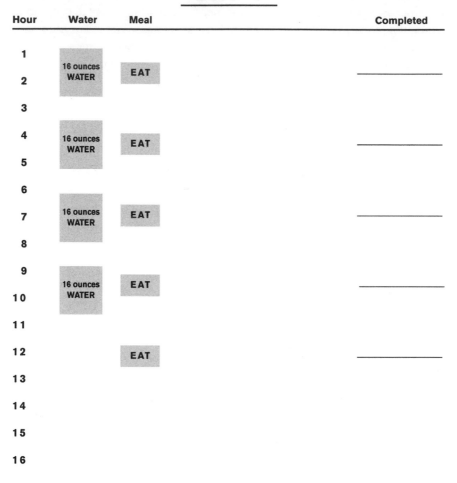

Hour	Water	Meal		Completed
1				
	16 ounces WATER	EAT		_____
2				
3				
4				
	16 ounces WATER	EAT		_____
5				
6				
7	16 ounces WATER	EAT		_____
8				
9				
	16 ounces WATER	EAT		_____
10				
11				
12		EAT		_____
13				
14				
15				
16				

Difficulties and Insights

_____

_____

_____

_____

_____

_____

BODY BILL

DAY 2

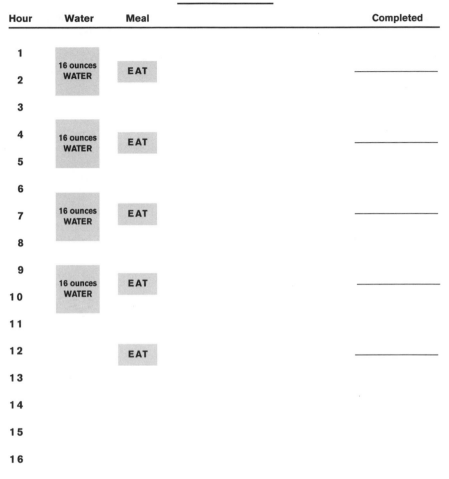

Hour	Water	Meal		Completed
1				
2	16 ounces WATER	EAT		_____
3				
4	16 ounces WATER	EAT		_____
5				
6				
7	16 ounces WATER	EAT		_____
8				
9	16 ounces WATER	EAT		_____
10				
11				
12		EAT		_____
13				
14				
15				
16				

Difficulties and Insights

_____

_____

_____

_____

_____

_____

BODY BILL

DAY 3

Hour	Water	Meal		Completed
1				
2	16 ounces WATER	EAT		_____
3				
4	16 ounces WATER	EAT		_____
5				
6				
7	16 ounces WATER	EAT		_____
8				
9				
10	16 ounces WATER	EAT		_____
11				
12		EAT		_____
13				
14				
15				
16				

Difficulties and Insights

_____

_____

_____

_____

_____

_____

BODY BILL

DAY 4

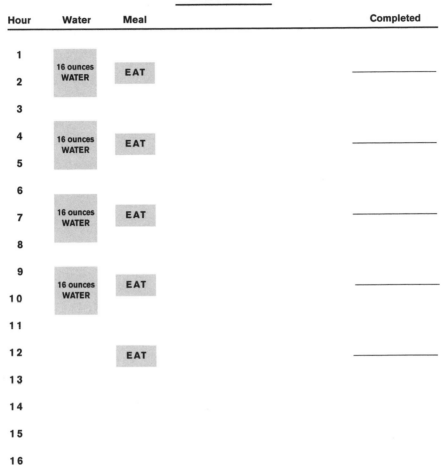

Hour	Water	Meal		Completed
1	16 ounces WATER	EAT		_____
2				
3				
4	16 ounces WATER	EAT		_____
5				
6				
7	16 ounces WATER	EAT		_____
8				
9	16 ounces WATER	EAT		_____
10				
11				
12		EAT		_____
13				
14				
15				
16				

Difficulties and Insights

BODY BILL

DAY 5

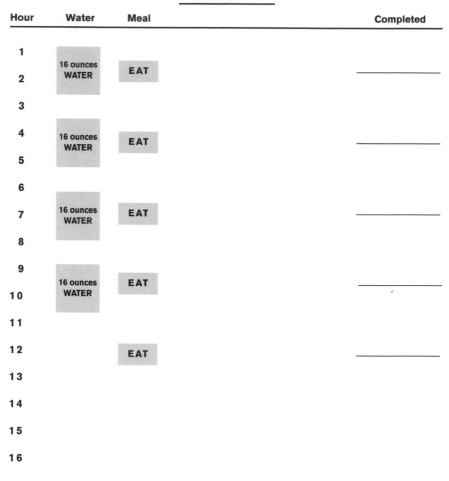

Hour	Water	Meal		Completed
1				
2	16 ounces WATER	EAT		_____
3				
4	16 ounces WATER	EAT		_____
5				
6				
7	16 ounces WATER	EAT		_____
8				
9				
10	16 ounces WATER	EAT		_____
11				
12		EAT		_____
13				
14				
15				
16				

Difficulties and Insights

_____

_____

_____

_____

_____

_____

BODY BILL

DAY 6

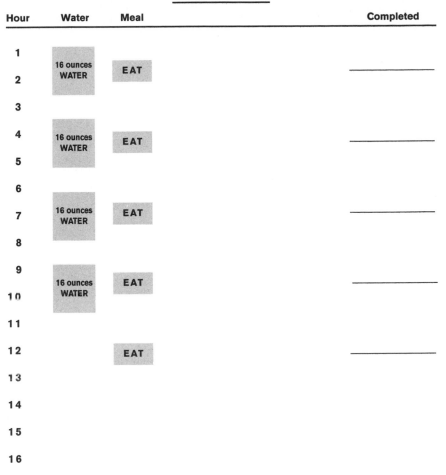

Hour	Water	Meal		Completed
1				
	16 ounces WATER	EAT		_____
2				
3				
4				
	16 ounces WATER	EAT		_____
5				
6				
7	16 ounces WATER	EAT		_____
8				
9				
	16 ounces WATER	EAT		_____
10				
11				
12		EAT		_____
13				
14				
15				
16				

Difficulties and Insights

_____

_____

_____

_____

_____

_____

BODY BILL

DAY 7

Hour	Water	Meal		Completed
1				
	16 ounces WATER	EAT		_____
2				
3				
4				
	16 ounces WATER	EAT		_____
5				
6				
7	16 ounces WATER	EAT		_____
8				
9				
	16 ounces WATER	EAT		_____
10				
11				
12		EAT		_____
13				
14				
15				
16				

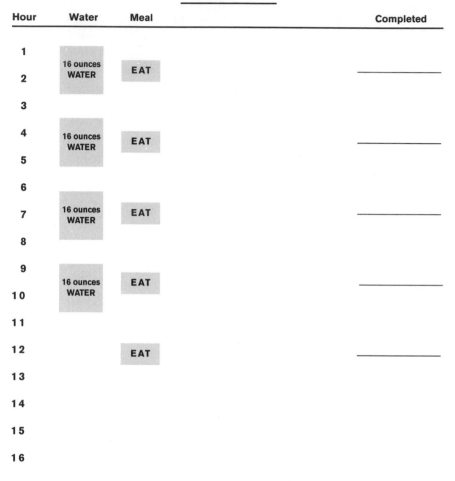

Difficulties and Insights

_____

_____

_____

_____

_____

_____

CHAPTER FIVE

STEP THREE

Equation for Perfect Portions— Size Does Matter

It is possible that by properly hydrating yourself and eating several meals at the same time every day, you have achieved the results you desired. However, it is much more likely that your eating program needs a few small adjustments to become the perfect equation for you.

Last week, you began the process of creating a new habit—a new way of eating. For the last seven days, you ate shortly after waking up, ate many small meals throughout the day, and finished your last meal around sunset. While this may have seemed quite simple when you read it, this small change to your lifestyle was the most difficult transition that you will have to make on this program.

By eating in this new way, you have begun the process of striking a balance in your nutritional program. It is a balancing act that will require small adjustments. Let's return to the car metaphor. For a moment, think of your body as a finely tuned car and think of food as if it were gasoline. That car can be the most expensive, most luxurious, and highest performance car ever made, but without gas in its tank, the car won't move. If you were on a coast-to-coast race, you would periodically need to refuel your car. You wouldn't want to carry extra fuel with you, because that extra weight would limit how fast you could go. You would want only enough fuel to get you to the next fuel stop—no more, no less. Eating is much the same. You need to eat to live. To live healthfully, to live with vitality, to have energy, you need to have just the right amount of food. When your tank is empty, you need to refuel. By putting the right amount of fuel in your tank at the right time, your engine will run at the highest levels of performance, and you will burn your fuel efficiently.

The greatest mistake that dieters make is eating too much or too little, and often we complicate our dilemma by doing both at the same time. When you eat too much, your body can use only a small percentage of that food and stores the rest away as fat to be used later. When you eat too little, your body believes itself to be starving, so it conserves its energy by using only the bare minimum energy to fuel your basic bodily functions and stores the rest away in your fat cells. Often, people make both of these mistakes at the same time. You may have waited too long to eat, so then you overeat to compensate for how hungry you are. If you are to have any hope of parting with the fat you have, it is essential that you eat enough to prevent the starvation-protection device from becoming active but not so much that your body cannot use all of the food to fuel activity and bodily functions.

Most of us, even the most disciplined eaters, overeat on occasion. It cannot be overemphasized: Overeating makes you fatter. Common sense alone should be all you need to understand how this happens, but there have been many studies that prove this fact scientifically. There also have been unexplained spikes in levels of obesity that pertain to the quantities of food consumed. Research has shown that the percentage of children who were overweight doubled over the last 30 years. From 1963 to 1980, these percentages stayed fairly level, but there was an enormous spike in the mid-1980s. The scientific community scrambled to come up with an explanation. Mysteriously, this spike in obesity also took place in adult populations, and this complicated the questions and really puzzled all the experts. There were no new foods introduced during this time period, it was determined that people were eating the same things as they were 10 years earlier, and there is no solid information to point to a cause. What was overlooked was the *amount* of food that was being consumed. In the mid-1980s, consumers of fast food were introduced to the concept of "supersizing." Positioned as a "value," consumers were given more food for their money, and as a consequence of supersizing, they got exactly what was promised—a bigger size. It's just too much food for your body to use! The majority of that extra-value meal will end up contained within your fat cells.

EATING CONSCIOUSNESS

This week you are adding another layer to your personal equation. From this point forward, you will continue to hydrate yourself as you did in week one, and you will continue to eat your meals at the same times you ate last week, but you will be striking a balance with the *amount* of food you eat. That balance is created by becoming conscious about what and how much food you are putting into your body. That balance is something that you will be honing and adjusting until you find the perfect way of eating. When you discover the perfect way of eating for you, you will have created your own personal equation. In creating your own personal equation, you will also have created a new lifestyle. When you combine your own personal equation with a new lifestyle, you can create a new you.

In creating the perfect way of eating, and developing a strategy to release stored fat, it is important to know what fat is, what fat does, and how fat accumulates. When you eat, your body uses the food as energy. You need that energy to keep your lungs breathing and your heart pumping, and to fuel physical activity. Your heart pumps blood throughout your body, and your blood carries nutrients to any other part of your body that is working. When you eat, your body uses only the food it needs at that very moment. If there is a surplus, your body breaks down the food and stores the essential ingredients it needs for fuel into your fat cells like a reserve fuel tank. In other words, if you eat more than your body needs, the surplus is stored within fat cells to be used later. To prevent this from happening, it is essential to learn how much food your body needs and how much is too much.

This week your goal is to learn the greatest secret of weight loss; the difference between eating until you feel satisfied and eating until you are full. Truly, this is the difference between eating to live and living to eat. Look at eating realistically. Your stomach, the actual organ in your body, is not large. With the exception of your spine, there are no bones in this area. The area between your belt and your rib cage is surrounded by muscle on all sides and is filled with the intestine, liver, gallbladder, and kidneys. Only a small portion of that area is devoted to your stomach. Your stomach can stretch and shrink, and when you have eaten a very large meal (like Thanksgiving dinner) it can grow to be the size of your head. But even at this size, your stomach is full of acids and other liquids, which are what break down the food you eat. Realistically, there is just not that much room in your stomach for food. All of us have a tendency to overeat. The lesson is that you do not have to eat very much to survive, and it really does not take much food to make you feel satisfied.

There are many benefits of eating enough to feel satisfied but not so much that you feel full. Think of how you feel after Thanksgiving dinner. Think of the feeling that just one more bite might make you burst. What happens after that meal? Getting up from the table and running around, doing errands or getting in some work are the farthest thoughts from your mind. Chances are you cannot wait to unfasten your pants and lounge or take a nap. For most of us, overeating is not a once-a-year phenomenon; it happens at almost every meal. If you feel sluggish, fatigued, or downright tired after meals, chances are that you are overeating. Physiologically, all of that food in the stomach needs digesting, and our digestive system requires increased circulation to and within our stomach and digestive organs to process that food. This in turn makes us less energetic than we would normally be. Now look at the opposite extreme. If you go too long between meals, you will have a tendency to gorge, to overeat, to eat until and even after you are full. Waiting too long to eat, and eating only when you are famished, prevents you from attaining your goal.

When we eat to a level of satisfaction rather than eating until we are full, we remain energized, focused, and balanced. Have you ever referred to anyone as "hungry"? What does that really mean? It certainly doesn't mean that he or she is malnourished. It means that the person is ready and eager, willing to give it his or her all. Couldn't we all be a little bit more "hungry"? Aren't these qualities that we should have more, not less, of? Much of being in this frame of mind, a mentality of readiness, has to do with having enough to be satisfied but not enough so that you are full. The human body operates most effectively on all levels when we are not overfed. Rate your level of hunger on a scale from 1 to 10, with 1 representing the way you would feel if you hadn't eaten for 24 hours, and 10 representing the way you feel after Thanksgiving dinner. If you could always remain at about 4, all of your systems would operate at an optimal level.

ADDICTED TO 4

Have you ever had a physiological reaction to the food you ate? People who have eaten sushi commonly refer to such a reaction as a "protein high." They feel energized, virile, and charged after eating. People who eat sugar-laden foods also get a similar reaction. They feel an increase of energy or a "sugar buzz." This feeling does not have to be attributed to a certain food or food group, rather, it is a feeling you can experience throughout the day. On the hunger scale of 1 to 10, if you can maintain your level of hunger at about 4, you can experience this intensified energy level all the time. Instead of reaching for a candy bar or other stimulant to induce this state, your level of "fullness" will begin to power you in a similar fashion. This natural "high" will become as addicting and as pleasurable as chocolate, but much more beneficial. Not only does this level of fullness create a physical state where all of your bodily functions are operating at optimum levels, but remaining at the fullness level of 4 also is a great service to maintaining if not reducing the amount of fat on your body. Staying at the level of 4 may be unfamiliar or mildly uncomfortable at first, but once you experience and sustain this level for a few days, it will become the place of balance between hungry and full where you feel your best. After a few days, you may feel so productive, so focused, that this becomes your level of choice.

Over the next week you will begin to learn how to eat enough so that your body has all the energy it needs to power you through the day, but not to eat too much so that your body stores away that excess food into your fat. The object of this exercise is to speed the metabolism to its highest possible rate, quickly and completely burning all the fuel we put into the furnace.

HOW MUCH IS ENOUGH?

While you are eating five meals per day, and eating at the same times every day, you can now create a guideline for how much food you eat at those meals. For each meal, you may choose any three foods. If you are craving a certain food, by all means have it! By choosing three different food groups, you will be getting basic nutritional requirements, such as protein, carbohydrate, and fruits and vegetables. Of course, keep your intake of fats and sugars at a minimum.

Some people fear that eating many meals will have the exact opposite effect of what they desire. The secret is in the size of your meals, and the size of each portion is the key to not overeating. This portion size is easy to estimate. For breakfast, lunch, and dinner, each of your three items should never be larger than the approximate size of your clenched fist. When looking at your fist, this size represents approximately one cup or 8 ounces of food (half that size represents approximately 4 ounces). Between breakfast and lunch and between lunch and dinner you should be eating a small snack. The snacks should be smaller than meals. The size can either be one fist-sized portion (a piece of fruit) or three palm-sized portions. Imagine that you were going to take a drink of water from a crystal clean lake. You would cup one hand and lift that amount of water to your lips. The amount of water that could be held in your hand would equal one portion size.

The goal is for you to be able to quickly determine portion sizes. Try some measurements for yourself using your favorite foods. Compare your "fist-sized" portion to the same amount in a measuring cup. Check to see how many ounces can fit into your palm. Just for fun, fill a bowl of cereal with the amount you would usually eat, and before you pour in the milk, use a measuring cup to determine how much cereal is in the bowl. By doing experiments such as these you can quickly estimate the amount of food on your plate.

Eating at least five meals per day, with each meal having appropriate portions, creates a sound nutritional program that allows you to reduce the amount of fat on your body, but it is essential that you strive to meet your basic nutritional requirements. The best information that science has to offer us on basic nutritional requirements is the American Food Guide Pyramid.[6] This food pyramid has been used for decades and is refined every few years. By following the suggestions set forth, you are taking the best advice of the American Medical Association, the United States Department of Health and Human Services, and the Centers for Disease Control.

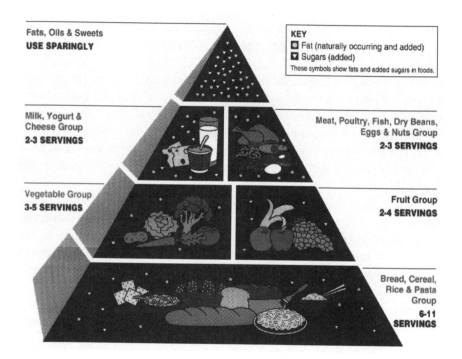

What Is a Serving?

Milk, Cheese, Yogurt:

1 cup of milk, 2 ounces of cheese, 8 ounces of yogurt

Meats, Poultry, Fish, Seafood, Dry Beans, Eggs, Nuts:

Amounts should total 2 to 3 ounces cooked lean meat
Count 1 egg or 2 tablespoons peanut butter as 1 ounce lean meat (about ⅓ portion)

Vegetables–Dark Green Leafy, Deep Yellow, Beans, Peas, Potatoes:

½ cup raw or cooked vegetables, 1 cup leafy greens, ¾ cup vegetable juice

Fruits:

A medium-size apple, banana, or orange; ½ grapefruit; a melon wedge; ¾ cup fruit juice; ½ cup berries; ¼ cup canned or dried fruit

Bread, Cereal, Rice, Pasta:

1 slice of bread; ½ hamburger bun or English muffin; a small roll, biscuit, or muffin; 3 or 4 small or 2 large crackers; ½ cup cooked cereal, rice, pasta; 1 ounce cold cereal

THE PROGRAM

This week, your five meals will have portion sizes. By limiting your portion sizes, you will not overeat, you will burn off all of the food you do eat to maintain bodily functions and to fuel activity, and you will never feel hungry.

1. Breakfast, lunch, and dinner should each be made up of at least three food groups found on the food guide pyramid. Portion sizes for each of these should not exceed the size of your clenched fist.
2. Eat two snacks per day: one between breakfast and lunch, and the other between lunch and dinner. The portion size for these snacks should either be one clenched fist, or three separate foods each with a portion size that could be held like water in your cupped hand.

WORKING THE EQUATION

Often we feel unsatisfied after a meal. You may feel that you "just need a few more bites." For you, it is the "little bit extra" that you would like to do without.

- Wait at least 20 minutes after eating before you have additional food.
- Drink a glass of water after your meal to feel "satisfied."

Perhaps you feel satisfied by a meal only after you have cleaned your plate. If this is the case, shift the circumstances. Instead of eating from a large dinner plate, eat your meals from a bread plate.

WHAT YOU CAN EXPECT THIS WEEK

This week you can expect to see results. Your body is relaxing its starvation-protection device, and by eating portions that are more appropriate, you may actually see 1½ to 2 pounds of fat loss as a result of a rock-solid nutritional program.

MAKING IT WORK

Modify

1. Make your snack something that is easy to take with you. "On-the-go" snacks like fruit, snack and meal-replacement bars, and protein or meal-replacement drinks are the easiest.
2. Wait at least 20 minutes after a meal to attain a feeling of satisfaction.

Substitute

1. Begin substituting healthy foods for sugary and fatty foods. Instead of a morning doughnut, have a bagel or toast. Switch from regular ice cream to fruit, low-fat or nonfat desserts.

2. Substitute any current late-night habits like drinking beer or eating regular chips with low-cal foods like diet drinks and baked chips.

Shift

1. Reduce or stop eating high-fat and high-sugar foods.
2. Add a salad or soup to your meal and cut down other foods accordingly.

YOUR BODY BILL

Just as in the previous chapters, it is important to check off a completed task. This week you must still drink at least four 16-ounce glasses of water each day, you must eat five times, and each of those meals should reflect the food groups. After your first day or two, again look over the food guide pyramid to see if you are meeting the suggested nutritional guidelines.

BODY BILL

DAY 1

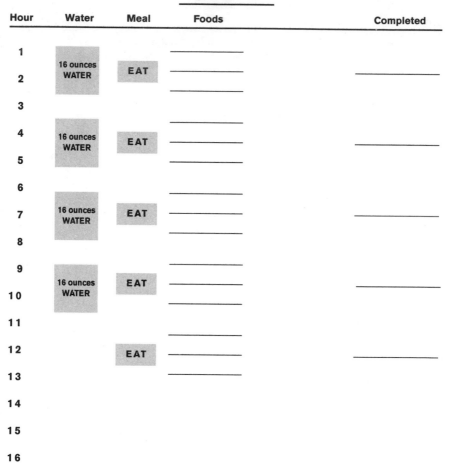

Hour	Water	Meal	Foods	Completed
1			_____	
2	16 ounces WATER	EAT	_____	_____
3			_____	
4			_____	
5	16 ounces WATER	EAT	_____	_____
6			_____	
7	16 ounces WATER	EAT	_____	_____
8			_____	
9			_____	
10	16 ounces WATER	EAT	_____	_____
11			_____	
12		EAT	_____	_____
13			_____	
14				
15				
16				

Difficulties and Insights

_____

_____

_____

_____

_____

_____

BODY BILL

DAY 2

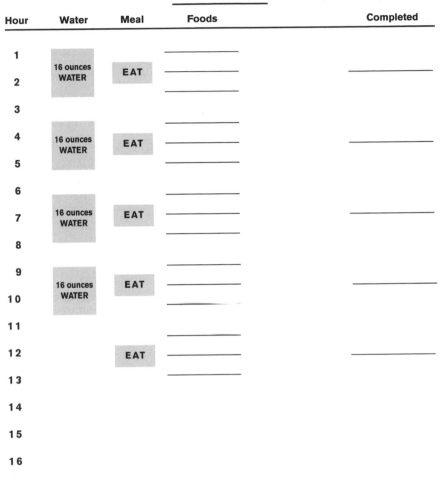

Hour	Water	Meal	Foods	Completed
1			_____	
2	16 ounces WATER	EAT	_____	_____
3			_____	
4	16 ounces WATER	EAT	_____	_____
5			_____	
6			_____	
7	16 ounces WATER	EAT	_____	_____
8			_____	
9			_____	
10	16 ounces WATER	EAT	_____	_____
11			_____	
12		EAT	_____	_____
13			_____	
14				
15				
16				

Difficulties and Insights

_____

_____

_____

_____

_____

_____

BODY BILL

DAY 3

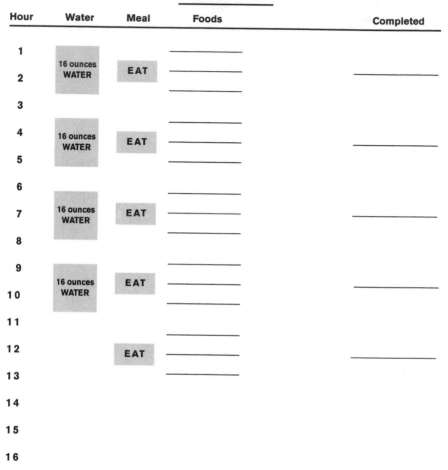

Hour	Water	Meal	Foods		Completed
1			———————		
2	16 ounces WATER	EAT	———————		———————
3			———————		
4			———————		
5	16 ounces WATER	EAT	———————		———————
6			———————		
7	16 ounces WATER	EAT	———————		———————
8			———————		
9			———————		
10	16 ounces WATER	EAT	———————		———————
11			———————		
12		EAT	———————		———————
13			———————		
14					
15					
16					

Difficulties and Insights

_____

_____

_____

_____

_____

_____

BODY BILL

DAY 4

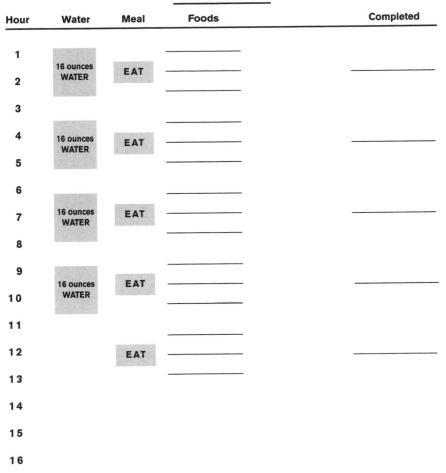

Hour	Water	Meal	Foods	Completed
1			_____	
	16 ounces WATER	EAT	_____	_____
2			_____	
3				
4			_____	
	16 ounces WATER	EAT	_____	_____
5			_____	
6			_____	
7	16 ounces WATER	EAT	_____	_____
8			_____	
9			_____	
	16 ounces WATER	EAT	_____	_____
10			_____	
11			_____	
12		EAT	_____	_____
13			_____	
14				
15				
16				

Difficulties and Insights

_____

_____

_____

_____

_____

_____

BODY BILL

DAY 5

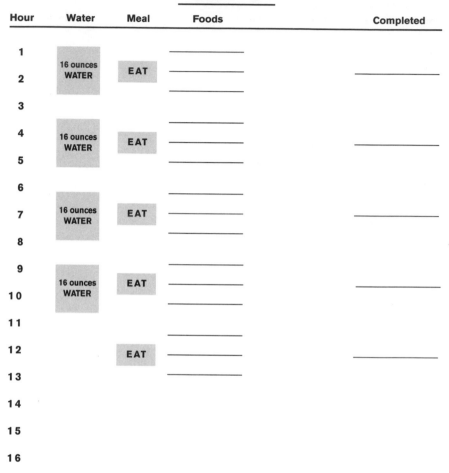

Hour	Water	Meal	Foods	Completed
1			_____	
2	16 ounces WATER	EAT	_____	_____
3			_____	
4			_____	
5	16 ounces WATER	EAT	_____	_____
6			_____	
7	16 ounces WATER	EAT	_____	_____
8			_____	
9			_____	
10	16 ounces WATER	EAT	_____	_____
11			_____	
12		EAT	_____	_____
13			_____	
14				
15				
16				

Difficulties and Insights

_____

_____

_____

_____

_____

_____

BODY BILL

DAY 6

Hour	Water	Meal	Foods	Completed
1			————	
2	16 ounces WATER	EAT	———— ————	————
3				
4			————	
5	16 ounces WATER	EAT	———— ————	————
6			————	
7	16 ounces WATER	EAT	————	————
8			————	
9			————	
10	16 ounces WATER	EAT	———— ————	————
11			————	
12		EAT	————	————
13			————	
14				
15				
16				

Difficulties and Insights

_____

_____

_____

_____

_____

_____

BODY BILL

DAY 7

Hour	Water	Meal	Foods		Completed
1			_____		
2	16 ounces WATER	EAT	_____		_____
3			_____		
4			_____		
5	16 ounces WATER	EAT	_____		_____
6			_____		
7	16 ounces WATER	EAT	_____		_____
8			_____		
9			_____		
10	16 ounces WATER	EAT	_____		_____
11			_____		
12		EAT	_____		_____
13			_____		
14					
15					
16					

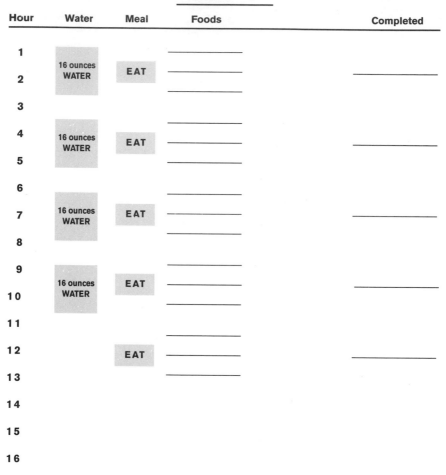

Difficulties and Insights

_____

_____

_____

_____

_____

_____

PART THREE

EQUATION

for

FAT LOSS

As you recall, the process of making a change in your life has five stages. You passed through the pre-contemplative and contemplative stage as you decided what to do about your situation. You passed through the action phase as you layered in several new patterns of behavior or habits and laid the foundation for a lean lifestyle. Without these alterations to your lifestyle, you cannot rid your body of fat, nor can you expect to maintain the results you are about to achieve.

Just by continuing to practice these new lifestyle habits you could get the results you desire. Over time, this new lifestyle could enable you to be 20 to 50 pounds lighter in a few years' time. For most of us, this sort of long-range projection is not in keeping with what we want. We want results, and we want them quickly. Part Three of this book adds another layer to the new lifestyle you are creating and accelerates the process of body-fat reduction.

Throughout the book we have made a number of analogies, two of which may help define what this next step actually does. In Part One, we made the analogy that creating the perfect nutritional program is much like setting up a scientific experiment. Before making an experiment, scientists have a hypothesis. In other words, they think they know what and why something is occurring, but they have to test that hypothesis by doing experiments. When scientists create an experiment, they follow a very exacting procedure so the findings of their experiments can be proved or disproved. This is often called a controlled test, where all of the baseline factors are the same, but one element is added to the test to conclude an outcome. Over the last three weeks, you have done exactly the same thing. You have made slight adjustments to your lifestyle, to better determine what will work for you. Then you added a piece of the puzzle, and then another. In Part Two, we made the analogy that getting rid of body fat is much like being a safe-cracker, and that you are trying to discover the correct combination in hopes of opening the door to a new future. You have, by creating a new lifestyle, success-fully determined three of the five numbers you need to enjoy the riches behind the door.

You are now drinking at least 64 ounces of water each day; you are eating several small meals per day, starting within one hour after you wake up and fin-ishing your last meal around sunset. You have limited the amount of fast food you are eating to a bare minimum. For each meal you are fulfilling your nutritional requirements by choosing foods from the food pyramid, and each is measured in fist- or palm-sized portions. You are eating meals at the exact same time each day. You are eating your food slowly, without distraction, and having at least one tradi-tional meal per day with family or friends. Like the scientist, you have made small adjustments to the experiment. You have learned a great deal about yourself and have done much to create a lifestyle that promotes a reduction of body fat. Like the safecracker, you are just two numbers away from hitting the jackpot.

This section of the book is about creating a strategy to meet your expecta-tions. It is a great thing to say, "I'd like to lose so many pounds of fat" or "I'd like to wear a smaller clothing size." It is even greater to come up with a strategy that will take you there. Part Three begins as a process of refining your food intake and creating a more exacting nutritional program, then takes you through the step-by-step process of burning off the energy stored within your fat cells.

CHAPTER SIX

STEP FOUR

Equation for Caloric Consumption

Think of this program as if you were building a house. You must first create a solid foundation to build on. Over the last three weeks you have done much work on this foundation: You have dug the hole, you have added reinforcements, and you have leveled off the ground. Now you are going to pour concrete in that area to make this foundation last.

Look at what you accomplished in only three weeks! You have started the process of developing the most beneficial habits that you could possibly have, and these habits will see you through to a dramatic physical transformation. These habits are really your secret weapon, the keys to the common patterns of behavior that most lean people have. By layering a routine that combines proper water intake with proper eating habits, you are living the way that the human body was designed for. You must be vigilant to maintain your water intake, you must be consistent in the timing of your meals, you must keep your portions small. When these new habits take hold, you will have made some tremendous changes to your lifestyle!

This is a critical point in your transformation. This is the point when most people give up or become impatient. You want to make changes to your physical appearance, and you want those changes to happen immediately, but the truth of the matter is that those changes cannot take place overnight. Instead of viewing the glass as half empty, you must see that the glass is half full. You have come a long way, and at this very moment, your body has reached a level of proper hydration and is starting to function better as a result. At this point, your body is becoming accustomed to being fed regularly and sufficiently, and is starting to process the food you eat in a completely new and more efficient manner. At this point, all of your food-related survival mechanisms are beginning to relax, they are beginning to trust that you will take care of your body and so they do not have to be on alert. As a result, your body is beginning the process of releasing what is held in storage. Your body can now begin to use the energy stored in your fat cells to power you through the day.

Still, you want results and you do not want to wait years for them. Part Three of this book teaches you to refine what you are eating so that you can begin to have those results. At this point you have come to some conclusions about what "proper eating" means to you, both in terms of the way you feel, and the amount of food your body actually needs. The greatest lesson you have learned is that your body can process only a certain amount of food at one time. If you have more than that amount, your body burns off only what it needs and then places all that "extra" food in your fat cells for later use. Unfortunately, the human body does not like to part with the energy held in reserve, and becoming more exacting in terms of how much you eat is the key to tapping into your reserve fuel tank. While limiting your portion sizes did much to bring about efficient use, a more exacting approach to food intake will enable you to burn the maximum amount of stored energy contained within your fat cells.

Determining how much food is enough requires that you add another layer to your behavior—one last building block before you can start the process of working your own personal equation for fat loss. Last week you defined "balance" as the place between hungry and full, but that was only to create a sense of comfort, a sense of satisfaction, and to complete the relaxation process for your starvation-protection device. If you want to burn off fuel from the reserve tank (your fat cells), there is another step. That next step is creating a numeric value for the food you eat, so that you can determine exactly how much is enough.

The question of "how much is enough" can be answered only by you. To assess how much you need, you simply place a numeric value on the foods you are eating. This numeric value is determined by the caloric value of food. To complete this next step in your transformation, you need to determine how many calories you need and regulate the amount of calories you are taking in.

In basic scientific terms, a calorie refers to energy. In the laboratory, one calorie is the amount of energy required to raise the temperature of one cubic centimeter of water by one degree. After this point caloric values become less exacting. To a large degree calories are estimates. Food, for instance, has a caloric value. In the laboratory a food will be incinerated in a closed container and scientists determine the "caloric value" of a food by the rise in temperature. They may do this experiment a hundred different times, and average out the differing results to come up with a number. That number, *on average*, represents a caloric value for that particular food. Like food, body fat also contains calories. *On average*, the scientists determined that a pound of body fat contains 3,500 calories. Your body fat may contain more or less, but each pound of body fat you have contains *approximately* 3,500 calories.

This number is an extremely important guideline for you and relates directly to what you are doing this week. You goal is not to lose random "weight," but to rid yourself of body fat. If a pound of body fat represents approximately 3,500 calories, it follows that if you reduce your caloric intake by this 3,500 calories, you can lose one pound of fat. Hidden in this fact is the real truth about weight loss and fat loss. You could simply starve yourself and easily create a caloric deficit, and most commercial "diets" do exactly that. However, an extreme reduction in calories does not guarantee that lost weight will actually come from stored fat. Again, it is counter-productive to starve yourself, as this will merely set off a chain reaction of starvation-protection mechanisms, which actually prevents a loss of fat. Eating in the manner you are currently eating is the safe and correct way to go about your transformation, as these many small meals disarm the starvation-protection device. Even though eating many small meals turns off starvation-protection mechanisms, and eating appropriately sized meals prevents you from storing any more fat, you must now reduce the caloric value of those meals to effect a reduction of fat.

Much like what you have done over the last three weeks, this process is a balancing act. This sense of balance must keep the starvation-protection device from becoming activated but not give the body all the food it needs. In reality, the balance you are striking this week will cause an imbalance. You will need to take in enough calories so that your body does not think it is starving but not enough to fuel your activity. To make up for this energy deficit, your body will have to call upon its reserve tank, your stored fat, for power. Striking this balance will require a little bit of strategy, and some simple discipline, but be assured that you are merely refining what you are currently doing.

Coming up with a winning strategy requires some basic understanding. The first and most elementary thing that you must define is how much food you need to prevent your starvation-protection device from becoming active. As part of this strategy you should determine how many calories you need each day. Just as there are scientifically based estimates regarding the caloric value of food, each individual requires a different number of calories each day. There are more exacting methods to determine this exact num-ber, processes that are cumbersome and complex, but over the years we have found a simple method to calculate an estimate for this number, and have found that it comes surprisingly close to scientifically based testing.

To determine how many calories you need each day, simply weigh yourself on the scale. Add a zero to the end of your weight. That is the total number of calories that you need to eat to maintain your weight. For example, if you weigh 150 pounds, you will burn off 1,500 calories per day if you are at rest. Technically this is called your "basal metabolic rate." If you merely get out of bed you burn even more calories. Just by tinkering around the house, reading the morning paper, cooking your meals, and performing routine household tasks, you would expend an additional 300 calories per day. How many meals are you eating each day? The answer should be five. So divide your total caloric intake by 5. If you divide 1,500 by 5, you find that you need to eat 300 calories at each meal to fulfill your daily requirement.

Try It for Yourself

1. You weigh _____ on the scale. Add a zero to the end of that number: _____. This is how many calories you need to eat each day.

2. You eat 5 times per day.

3. Total calories per day _____ ÷ 5 = _____ calories per meal.

Now that you have determined how many calories you need to eat each day, and the number of calories you should have in each meal, it is essential that you know how many calories you must ingest before you activate your starvation-protection device. Generally this is a slippery slope, and this level of caloric reduction is different for every individual. In most cases, you could reduce your caloric intake up to 20 percent without activating your starvation-protection device, however this is not true of everyone. Therefore, we suggest that you reduce your caloric consumption by only 10 percent. This means that if you weigh 150 pounds, you need 1,500 calories just to maintain bodily functions. So you could safely reduce your caloric intake by 10 percent or (150 calories) before your starvation-protection device is activated. This works out to 1,350 calories per day and 270 calories per meal.

1. You need _____ calories per day (add a zero to your weight on the scale). This is your ideal caloric intake. Reduce this number by 10 percent.

2. Your ideal caloric intake _____ × .10 = _____. This represents your caloric minimum. If you eat any less than this amount you may

activate your starvation-protection device and limit the amount of

fuel that can be called upon from stored fat.

WHERE DO MY CALORIES COME FROM?

In the last chapter you began eating in a way that fulfilled your nutritional requirements by choosing foods from the food pyramid. The daily portions were specified so that you could meet the basic nutritional requirements of a balanced diet. Like last week, you will continue to choose three foods from the food pyramid for each meal. Like last week, you will continue to eat similarly sized meals. Unlike last week, you will further define your portion sizes by giving them a caloric value.

Essentially what you did last week was to use your first or your palm to determine your portion size. These guidelines gave you the ability to recognize and create more appropriate portions, and also to equate your hand as a measuring tool. The two portion sizes that were suggested were your clenched fist and your cupped palm. In simple terms, your fist represented approximately 1 cup, and your cupped palm represented approximately ⅓ cup. Because all of us have differing hand sizes, you now need to create a numeric value for the size of your hands, and create an easy method to tally your calories. Most calorie counters list a food and provide a corresponding caloric value to a portion size. For instance, oatmeal has approximately 110 calories per cup, cheddar cheese has approximately 110 calories per ounce, 4 ounces of shellfish contain approximately 110 calories, and olive oil contains approximately 110 calories per tablespoon. This week you will check simple hand measurements against the actual portion sizes to determine caloric values for the foods you eat. In other words, pour a fist-size portion of cereal into your bowl and, before you add milk, pour that cereal into a measuring cup to determine how close your "approximation size" is to the actual size of the portion you are trying to guesstimate. By doing this regularly throughout the week, you will get a much better idea of how much food equals how many calories. In reality, after about a week you will be able to eyeball a plate of food and determine how many calories are on the plate. The point of this exercise is simply to learn how to equate caloric values to the food you see before you.[7]

To better determine how many calories you are eating requires you to equate a specific portion of food with a specific number of calories. You can purchase calorie counter books at any bookstore, but the truth of the matter is that you really need only a condensed list. Most of us eat from a fairly limited menu. What follows is a list of the foods that make up each food group and an appropriate corresponding caloric value.[8]

EQUATION FOR ESTIMATING PORTION SIZES

1 cup = 1 fist   ⅓ cup = 1 cupped hand (palm)

1 teaspoon = 1 thumb tip (tip of thumb to knuckle)

1 tablespoon = 3 thumb tips

1 ounce of cheese = 1 thumb

1 ounce of nuts = 1 cupped palmful

1 ounce of chips or pretzels = 2 cupped palmfuls

6 ounces of chicken (breast) = 1 fist

4 ounces of fish = 1 cupped hand

FATS, OILS, SWEETS

FATS AND OILS	PORTION	CALORIES
Bacon, salt pork	2 slices	60
Butter	1 tbsp.	100
Cream cheese	2 tbsp.	100
Lard	1 tbsp.	115
Margarine	1 tbsp.	100
Mayonnaise	1 tbsp.	100
Mayonnaise-type salad dressing	1 tbsp.	70
Salad dressing	2 tbsp.	130
Shortening	1 tbsp.	115
Sour cream	2 tbsp.	60
Vegetable oil	1 tbsp.	120
Olive oil	1 tbsp.	120
SWEETS	**PORTION**	**CALORIES**
Hard candy	3 pieces	70
Frosting (icing)	2 tbsp.	130
Fruit drinks	8 fl. oz.	125

SWEETS	PORTION	CALORIES
Gelatin desserts	½ cup	80
Honey	1 tbsp.	60
Jam, jelly	1 tbsp.	50
Maple syrup	¼ cup	210
Marmalade	1 tbsp.	60
Molasses	1 tbsp.	60
Frozen fruit bar	1 bar	50
Sherbet	½ cup	120
Soft drinks and colas	8 fl. oz.	100
Sugar, white	1 tbsp.	46
Sugar, brown	1 oz.	107

ALCOHOLIC BEVERAGES	PORTION	CALORIES
Beer	12 fl. oz.	145
Liquor	1 fl. oz.	65
Wine	1 fl. oz.	25

DAIRY	PORTION	CALORIES
Milk, low-fat (1%)	8 fl. oz.	100
Milk, low-fat (2%)	8 fl. oz.	120
Milk, skim	8 fl. oz.	85
Milk, whole	8 fl. oz.	150
Half and half	1 tbsp.	20
Nondairy creamer	1 tbsp.	20
Nondairy creamer with flavor	1 tbsp.	40
Buttermilk	1 tbsp.	25
Cottage cheese, low-fat	½ cup	120
Cheddar cheese	1 oz.	110
Swiss cheese	1 oz.	90
Cheese spread	2 tbsp.	100
Yogurt, low-fat plain	8 oz.	150
Yogurt, fat-free	8 oz.	110
Yogurt, nonfat frozen	½ cup	100

DAIRY	PORTION	CALORIES
Yogurt, fruited	6 oz.	180
Ice cream	½ cup	150
Pudding made with skim milk	4 oz.	160

MEATS, FISH, EGGS	PORTION	CALORIES
Beef*	4 oz.	300
Chicken breast*	4 oz.	195
Fish*	4 oz.	160
Pork*	4 oz.	325
Lamb*	4 oz.	300
Ham*	4 oz.	330
Shellfish*	4 oz.	112
Turkey*	4 oz.	180
Veal*	4 oz.	215
Lunch meat	2 oz.	160
Sausage	1 link	120
Beans, dried	¼ cup	160
Eggs	1 large	75
Nuts and seeds	1 oz.	160
Peanut butter	2 tbsp.	200
Tofu	3 oz.	60

*All portions cooked

VEGETABLES

DARK GREEN LEAFY	PORTION	CALORIES
Mixed greens	½ cup	30
Broccoli	½ cup	10
Chicory	½ cup	20
Collard greens	½ cup	5
Dandelion	½ cup	15
Endive	½ cup	5

DARK GREEN LEAFY	PORTION	CALORIES
Escarole	½ cup	5
Kale	½ cup	20
Mustard greens	½ cup	10
Lettuce	½ cup	5
Spinach	½ cup	5
Turnip greens	½ cup	10
Watercress	½ cup	2

DEEP YELLOW	PORTION	CALORIES
Carrots	½ cup	25
Pumpkin	½ cup	15
Sweet potato	½ cup	80
Squash, winter	½ cup	50

STARCHY	PORTION	CALORIES
Corn	½ cup	90
Green peas	½ cup	60
Hominy (grits)	¼ cup	140
Potato	½ cup	70
Rutabaga	½ cup	25
Taro	½ cup	30

DRY BEANS AND PEAS (LEGUMES)	PORTION	CALORIES
Black beans	½ cup	115
Black-eyed peas	½ cup	100
Chickpeas	½ cup	135
Kidney beans	½ cup	112
Lentils	½ cup	115
Lima beans	½ cup	104
Mung beans	½ cup	110
Navy beans	½ cup	129
Pinto beans	½ cup	120
Split peas	½ cup	115

OTHER VEGETABLES	PORTION	CALORIES
Artichoke	1	60
Asparagus	4 spears	15
Bean and alfalfa sprouts	1 cup	10
Beets	½ cup	30
Cabbage	½ cup	10
Cauliflower	½ cup	13
Celery	½ cup	10
Cucumber	1	40
Eggplant	½ cup	15
Green beans	½ cup	20
Green pepper	1	20
Lettuce	1 head	20
Mushrooms	½ cup	10
Okra	½ cup	20
Onions	½ cup	30
Radishes	½ cup	10
Snow Peas	½ cup	70
Tomato	½ cup	20
Turnips	½ cup	15
Vegetable juices	8 fl. oz.	60
Zucchini	½ cup	15

FRUIT	PORTION	CALORIES
Apple	1 medium	80
Apricot	3 medium	50
Asian Pear	1 medium	100
Blueberries	½ cup	40
Cantaloupe	½ melon	95
Citrus juice	8 fl. oz.	140
Cherries	10 medium	50
Cranberries	½ cup	25
Dates	10	230
Fig	1 large	50

FRUIT	PORTION	CALORIES
Guava	1 medium	45
Grapes	10 medium	15
Grapefruit	½ medium	45
Honeydew	½ cup	30
Kiwi	1 medium	45
Lemon	1 medium	20
Mango	½ cup	55
Nectarine	1 medium	65
Orange	1 medium	70
Papaya	½ cup	25
Passion fruit	1 medium	20
Peach	1 medium	40
Pear	1 medium	100
Plantain	3 oz.	100
Pineapple	½ cup	40
Plum	1 medium	35
Prunes	10	200
Raisins	¼ cup	110
Raspberries	½ cup	30
Rhubarb	½ cup	15
Strawberries	½ cup	25
Tangerine	1 medium	35
Watermelon	½ cup	25

GRAINS, PASTA, RICE

WHOLE GRAIN	PORTION	CALORIES
Brown rice*	1 cup	230
Buckwheat*	¼ cup	150
Bulgur*	¼ cup	150
Corn tortillas	3 whole	140
Graham crackers	8	130
Granola	½ cup	190
Oatmeal	1 cup	109

WHOLE GRAIN	PORTION	CALORIES
Popcorn	2 tbsp. (uncooked)	150
Pumpernickel bread	1 slice	80
Ready-to-eat cereal	¾ cup	130
Rye bread	1 slice	80
Whole wheat bread	1 slice	70
Whole wheat pasta*	1 cup	175

ENRICHED GRAIN	PORTION	CALORIES
Bagel	½	100
Cornmeal*	¼ cup	130
Crackers	5	70
English muffin	1	140
Farina*	1 cup	115
Flour tortilla	1	130
French bread	1 slice	140
Hamburger and hot dog bun	1	135
Italian bread	2 slices	120
Macaroni*	1 cup	200
Noodle*	1 cup	210
Pancakes and Waffles	2 pieces	200
Pretzels	1 oz.	110
White rice*	¼ cup	150
Spaghetti*	1 cup	200
White bread	1 slice	80

*All portions cooked

GRAIN PRODUCTS WITH MORE FAT OR SUGAR	PORTION	CALORIES
Biscuit	1	140
Cake (unfrosted)	⅛ cake	200
Cookie	1	80
Cornbread	⅕ of a 10-inch pan	160
Croissant	1	140

GRAIN PRODUCTS WITH MORE FAT OR SUGAR	PORTION	CALORIES
Danish	1	130
Doughnut (plain)	1	170
Muffin/Scone	1	160
Tortilla Chips	1 oz.	150

THE PROGRAM

1. Step on the scale. Add a zero to the end of your weight.
   That is the amount of calories you need each day.
2. Divide the number of calories you need each day by 5.
   That is the amount of calories you need for each meal.
3. You should be able to reduce your caloric intake by 10 percent without setting off your starvation-protection device. If you weigh 120 pounds or less, DO NOT eat less than 1,200 calories per day.
4. Throughout the week compare the hand measurements you used last week with actual cup, ounce, teaspoon, and tablespoon measurements.
5. Add up your calories for every meal and tally them up at the end of the day. Limit your intake to the calories you need each day, and do not reduce your intake more than 10 percent below that level.

WORKING THE EQUATION

By the end of the week, you should be able to look at a food and determine how many calories it contains with only a very small margin of error. This is a tool that you are developing, and the more you can measure and weigh your food against your hand-size guideline, the easier and more second-nature this process will become for you.

WHAT YOU CAN EXPECT THIS WEEK

You will, without doubt, create a loss of body fat by the end of this week. How great that result is depends on two factors: the amount of calories you are eliminating (10 percent) and your level of activity. By adding a zero to the end of your weight you have determined exactly how many calories you need each day. If you reduce that number by 10 percent and maintain your present level of activity this could be the potential outcome: If you are disabled, ill, or do not get out of bed, you might lose up to ½ pound of body fat. If you are relatively inactive or stay at home, you could lose up to one pound of body fat this week. If you are moderately active, you could lose up to 1½ pounds of body fat this week. If you are extremely active, you could lose a little over 2 pounds of body fat in just 7 days.

BODY BILL

DAY 1

Hour	Water	Meal	Foods	Calories	Completed
1			_____	_____	
	16 ounces WATER	EAT	_____	_____	_____
2			_____	_____	
3			_____	_____	
4			_____	_____	
	16 ounces WATER	EAT	_____	_____	_____
5			_____	_____	
6			_____	_____	
7	16 ounces WATER	EAT	_____	_____	_____
8			_____	_____	
9			_____	_____	
	16 ounces WATER	EAT	_____	_____	_____
10			_____	_____	
11			_____	_____	
12		EAT	_____	_____	_____
13			_____	_____	
14					
15					
16					

Difficulties and Insights

_____

_____

_____

_____

_____

_____

BODY BILL

DAY 2

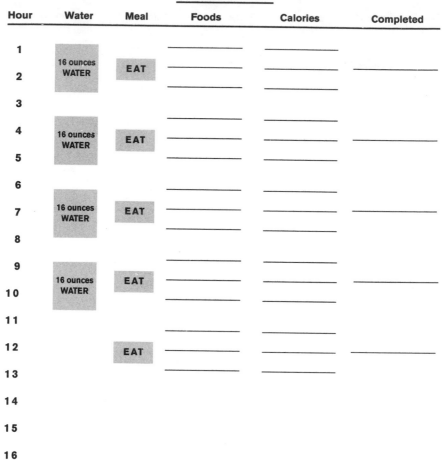

Hour	Water	Meal	Foods	Calories	Completed
1					
	16 ounces WATER	EAT			
2					
3					
4					
	16 ounces WATER	EAT			
5					
6					
7	16 ounces WATER	EAT			
8					
9					
	16 ounces WATER	EAT			
10					
11					
12		EAT			
13					
14					
15					
16					

Difficulties and Insights

_____

_____

_____

_____

_____

_____

BODY BILL

DAY 3

Hour	Water	Meal	Foods	Calories	Completed
1			_____	_____	
2	16 ounces WATER	EAT	_____	_____	_____
3			_____	_____	
4	16 ounces WATER	EAT	_____	_____	_____
5			_____	_____	
6			_____	_____	
7	16 ounces WATER	EAT	_____	_____	_____
8			_____	_____	
9			_____	_____	
10	16 ounces WATER	EAT	_____	_____	_____
11			_____	_____	
12		EAT	_____	_____	_____
13			_____	_____	
14					
15					
16					

Difficulties and Insights

_____

_____

_____

_____

_____

_____

BODY BILL

DAY 4

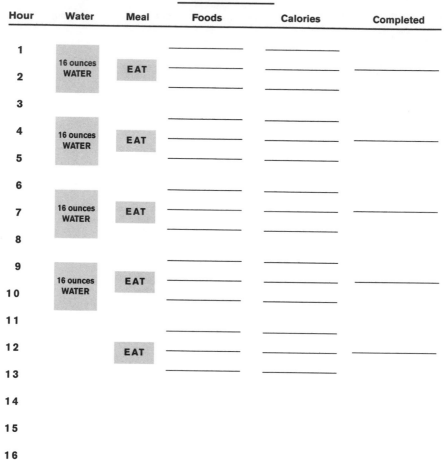

Hour	Water	Meal	Foods	Calories	Completed
1					
2	16 ounces WATER	EAT			
3					
4					
5	16 ounces WATER	EAT			
6					
7	16 ounces WATER	EAT			
8					
9					
10	16 ounces WATER	EAT			
11					
12		EAT			
13					
14					
15					
16					

Difficulties and Insights

_____

_____

_____

_____

_____

_____

BODY BILL

DAY 5

Hour	Water	Meal	Foods	Calories	Completed
1			_____	_____	
	16 ounces WATER	EAT	_____	_____	_____
2			_____	_____	
3					
4			_____	_____	
	16 ounces WATER	EAT	_____	_____	_____
5			_____	_____	
6			_____	_____	
7	16 ounces WATER	EAT	_____	_____	_____
8			_____	_____	
9			_____	_____	
	16 ounces WATER	EAT	_____	_____	_____
10			_____	_____	
11			_____	_____	
12		EAT	_____	_____	_____
13			_____	_____	
14					
15					
16					

Difficulties and Insights

_____

_____

_____

_____

_____

_____

BODY BILL

DAY 6

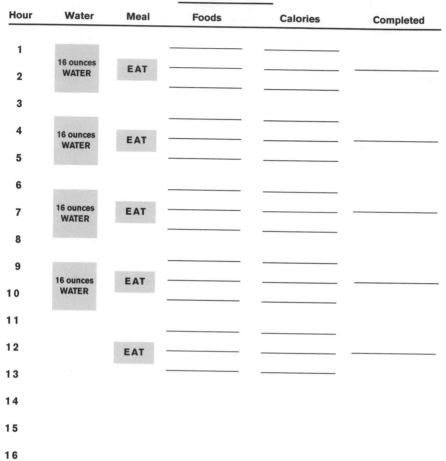

Hour	Water	Meal	Foods	Calories	Completed
1					
2	16 ounces WATER	EAT			
3					
4					
5	16 ounces WATER	EAT			
6					
7	16 ounces WATER	EAT			
8					
9					
10	16 ounces WATER	EAT			
11					
12		EAT			
13					
14					
15					
16					

Difficulties and Insights

_____

_____

_____

_____

_____

_____

BODY BILL

DAY 7

Hour	Water	Meal	Foods	Calories	Completed
1			_____	_____	
2	16 ounces WATER	EAT	_____	_____	_____
3			_____	_____	
4	16 ounces WATER	EAT	_____	_____	_____
5			_____	_____	
6			_____	_____	
7	16 ounces WATER	EAT	_____	_____	_____
8			_____	_____	
9			_____	_____	
10	16 ounces WATER	EAT	_____	_____	_____
11			_____	_____	
12		EAT	_____	_____	_____
13			_____	_____	
14					
15					
16					

Difficulties and Insights

_____

_____

_____

_____

_____

_____

CHAPTER SEVEN

STEP FIVE

Equation for Accelerating Fat Loss

Over the last weeks, you have added layer upon layer of positive habits to create a winning strategy that activated your body's natural fat-ridding abilities. You have been drinking at least 64 ounces of water a day, and that is now a habit that you have successfully developed and incorporated into your life. By the end of this week, you will have formed a habit of eating at least five times per day, starting within an hour after waking and stopping around sunset. You have refined your portion sizes, first by comparing them to your open or closed hand, and then by defining the caloric content of those portions. This behavior will be solidified as the new habit of eating only the calories you actually need, becomes yet another layer in your strategic arsenal.

By creating new habits or behaviors, you are creating a foundation on which to build your physical transformation. Again, these adjustments are minor, painless, and simple. No matter how small these adjustments seem, they will have an almost miraculous effect on your ability to rid your body of fat, to raise your energy level, and to improve your overall health. You are creating a foundation for sweeping and profound change to occur! It is essential to incorporate this foundation into your lifestyle, and you must be consistent with these new habits for the next 12 months to ensure that your physical transformation is as dramatic as you would like it to be and also to sustain your achievements throughout your life.

As you solidify this foundation, you disarm your survival mechanisms. As your body stores less of what you eat (accelerated metabolism), you now have the opportunity of using up what has been stored. This is an opportunity that you should not miss. Burning off what is stored in fat or energy depots is really the process of ridding yourself of unwanted body fat. Over the last four weeks you have given your body the go-ahead, the permission to use stored fat as fuel. With your newly built foundation in place you can create a specific strategy to call upon stored fat more and more frequently. This is the equation for accelerating your fat loss.

In the last chapter, you determined how much food your body needs. This is your personal baseline. This number reflects how many calories, or how much energy, you need just to maintain your basic bodily functions. To power additional activity, your body calls on stored fat for fuel. The process of ridding your body of fat is the fine art of using stored fat to fuel activity. This fine art is a balancing act, and to strike the perfect balance, you must employ activity as a method to get the results you desire.

This equation is simple to explain and even easier to understand and apply. In very simple terms, the equation is exactly like a seesaw—on one side is "calories in" and on the other side is "calories out." "Calories in" is what you eat, and "calories out" is the energy you expend. If you eat more calories than you burn off, you gain fat. If the seesaw is balanced, meaning you burn off as many calories as you take in, you maintain your weight. If you expend more calories than you eat, you call upon stored fat to fuel your activity and consequently rid yourself of fat and weight. The Equation simply places a numeric value on the calories you take in and the calories you burn off. The Equation is just that . . . an equation. It is as simple as 1 + 1 = 2. This chapter will provide the necessary tools to use The Equation for your own unique situation.

Earlier we stated that losing weight (fat) is extremely simple: Eat less and/or do more of the same activity you are already doing. Everyone who has ever lost weight has done one or the other or both. Whether they knew it or not, they used this equation. People engage in a physical activity like walking or jogging or some other form of exercise, and they lose weight. Other people go on a "diet," no matter what form, and invariably reduce the number of calories they take in. Again, no matter what diet you use, the number of calories you ingest is reduced, and common sense as well as science dictate that you will lose weight. It is that simple. You don't have to eat cabbage soup, or live exclusively on grapefruit, or eat only protein. When you reduce your calories, you lose weight, fat, and inches.

The point is that you can work The Equation to your own level of comfort and create a program that is more of a lifestyle choice than a restrictive regimen. When you incorporate The Equation into your lifestyle, you don't have to go on a new diet every six months. Once you begin to work The Equation, you are always in it, you are always enjoying the benefits, you are always seeing, realizing, and enjoying the result. The Equation simply provides a guideline so that your reduction is safe, effective, and scientifically sound. These guidelines are crucial. There are scientific limits to how far you can go and how hard you can push. These limits are dictated by the physiological response of the human body. There are only two basic guidelines for The Equation: calories in and calories out.

REDUCING CALORIES IN

You can tip the seesaw toward "calories out" and rid your body of fat simply by reducing your caloric intake. In the last chapter, you defined how many calories you must have to fuel your basic bodily functions. You did this by adding a zero to the end of your weight. This is exactly how many calories you need at rest. If you do any extra activity, you burn more calories and consequently are able to tap into your fat storage depot to fuel that activity. Last week, we have to assume that you at least got out of bed, which means that you created a calorie deficit. Over the course of the day, you expended at least 300 calories, meaning that over the course of the week you burned 2,100 calories. For this reason, there is no doubt that you lost weight on the scale, and the weight you lost came primarily from stored fat.

Last week, you also determined that there is a limit to how much you can reduce your caloric intake. We suggested that you can reduce your caloric intake by only 10 percent. If you reduce the total number of calories you eat each day by more than 20 percent, you certainly create a drastic caloric reduction. When you drastically reduce your caloric intake, you activate your starvation-protection device. If you have ever used a diet center, a diet from a magazine, or any other commercial diet not designed specifically for you, chances are that it involved a drastic reduction in total calories. In all probability, this drastic caloric reduction had some effect on your weight but little effect on your appearance. In other words, if you just used the diet, without any additional physical activity, you probably lost "weight." However, the weight you lost was in water, muscle, and bone density, but very little fat. As soon as you went back to eating as you did before the "diet," you put on all the "weight" you lost plus a little bit more. In reality, because you lost muscle and bone density on the diet, you ended up with a higher percentage of body fat than you had before you went on the diet. By reducing your caloric intake by more than 20 percent, you will not get the results you desire. In fact, you may get the exact opposite result than the one you are looking for.

INCREASING CALORIES OUT

In the last chapter, you may have read a cautionary note about people weighing less than 120 pounds. It was suggested that one should never decrease their total caloric intake below 1,200 calories, and for people in this category, there is another option to weight and fat loss. This option is one we should all take advantage of.

If you can reduce your caloric intake by only a relatively small percentage, you may find it necessary to tip the scales a little farther toward the "calories out" side of the seesaw. Again, losing fat, weight, and inches is as simple as burning off more calories than you take in. Therefore, by just doing more of the activities you are already doing, or even by creating a moderate exercise routine for yourself, you will be able to meet your goals easily and effortlessly.

We are built to burn off calories. We burn these calories continuously.[9] The goal is to be conscious about how you are burning off these calories and to create a method and accounting system to add up the calories you are burning. Each hour you are awake and walking around the house you are burning calories. If it is over 85° degrees outside, or extremely humid, you burn more calories to stay cool. If you are outside and it is below freezing, you burn more calories than normal to keep your body warm. In truth, you are burning calories all the time. During the course of an average day, most of us who are not extremely active, have physically demanding jobs, or who do not exercise will burn approximately 300 calories. With a little effort, you can burn even more.[10]

If you do yard work, you can rake the leaves more often. If you golf, you can walk the course rather than ride in a cart. If you work in an office building, you can walk up the stairs rather than ride the elevator. If you go out to lunch, you can walk to and from the restaurant. If you have a dog, you can walk it more frequently than you do now. If you use a snowblower for the sidewalk, you can use a shovel instead. If you take walks, you can increase your pace or extend the walk a longer distance. If you want to take up a sport or new activity, by all means do so! The incredible thing about activity is that everything you do counts in your equation. Activity is an aggregate, meaning that if you walk up the stairs, or to lunch, or a few miles around the neighborhood in the evening, all of that activity is added together. It all adds up on the "calories out" side of the seesaw.

USING THE EQUATION

We have set up a mathematical system for The Equation, so you can determine what you need to do each day and then each week to achieve your goal. This mathematical system has been tested for years, and it is the mechanism that enabled all the celebrity transformations to occur like clockwork.

This mathematical system is not an extravagant formula, but a point system that is much more like a credit card statement or your checkbook ledger, and it just adds another layer to what you have already been doing. Throughout the book, you have been filling in worksheets or body bills. This week you are given a point system with two columns: debits and credits. Both credits and debits are based on calories. When using The Equation, think of "calories in" as debits. These debits are like purchases, or money going out. Think of eating less, activity, and exercise as credits. These credits are a positive force that reduces your debt burden, or better yet, think of it as money coming into your account. Credits are something you want to attain, and by using The Equation, credits will be the currency of your transformation.

You can accumulate credits in two different ways: reduce the number of calories you are eating or increase your activity. Each activity you do is equated with a certain number of credits. All the various activities you do add up, and at the end of the day, you see these credits reflected on your body bill.

Again, these credits are based on calories. These numbers can get too high and too cumbersome, so we've simplified the math a little bit, so you do not need an accountant to add up your body bill. You have already determined what your total caloric intake for each day is, that you need those calories for a normal day, and that you burn those calories off for normal body functions. This is zero, your starting point. If you reduce your caloric intake by 100 calories, you get 1 credit. If you walk or run one mile, you burn 100 calories, and this also counts as 1 credit. In other words, you can either reduce your caloric intake by a small percentage or exercise to burn off extra calories, and for every 100 calories, you are awarded 1 credit.

The goal is to burn off more calories than you take in to facilitate a reduction in fat. There are two basic strategies to do this: eat fewer calories, or expend more calories through activity. We suggest that you do both. If you ran a marathon, you would burn off approximately 2,600 calories. If you ate a McDonald's quarter-pounder with cheese, a super-sized large fries, and large cola, you would have ingested about 2,600 calories. If you ran a marathon and only ate that meal on the same day, your points would equal out and you would be back at zero. But since you don't run a marathon every day, the simplest solution is to avoid foods with high caloric value, but this will be successful for you only to a certain extent. The better strategy is to reduce your caloric intake as much as you can within these guidelines, and partake in more of the activity you are already doing or a new form of exercise to tip the scales toward calories out.

It is important to understand how you can accumulate credits to tip the seesaw toward calories out. In your daily life, you can do many things to burn off calories. If you rake leaves or shovel snow for 30 minutes, you burn off 100 calories and receive 1 credit. If you walk briskly or run one mile, you burn off 100 calories and get 1 credit for your effort. If you walk the golf course instead of driving a cart, and play 18 holes, you get 1 credit. If you swim half a mile, you burn 100 calories and get 1 credit. If you walk up 20 flights of stairs, you get 1 credit. If you lift weights for 30 minutes you get 3 credits. If you use the StairMaster or elliptical trainer at the gym for one hour, you might accumulate 6 or 7 credits.

The objective becomes clear. The more credits you accumulate, the more fat you lose. If one credit represents 100 calories, and 1 pound of body fat contains approximately 3,500 calories, for every 35 credits you accumulate you lose 1 pound of fat. However, *there is a limit to how much you can reduce your weight and how much you can reduce your caloric intake.* First and foremost, on average you can safely lose 2 pounds of fat per week. In other words, you can and should accumulate a *maximum* of 70 credits per week. This does not mean that you might not lose more than that in a given week, but if you lose much more than 2½ pounds of fat per week, research tells us that you are less likely to be able to keep it off. If you are averaging more than 2½ pounds per week over a month or two, it may indicate that you are pushing The Equation too hard. The harder you drive your transformation, the greater the danger of stopping your physical transformation. Please proceed slowly and surely. If you lost only 1 pound per week, over the course of a year that is 52 pounds. If you lost only half a pound per week, that still totals 26 pounds in a year. You have the luxury of time, so afford yourself and your transformation the time you need to ensure that your results will last forever.

INCORPORATING ACTIVITY INTO YOUR LIFESTYLE

Just as you incorporated water into your day and made it part of your new lifestyle, you should begin to look at the activities you currently do as a foundation to build upon. As you can see, physical activity is an ideal way to tip the scales toward the calories out side of The Equation. There is no limit to how many credits you can accumulate by engaging in physical activity. Used as a strategy to reduce fat, activity is your greatest ally. Activity, more specifically regular exercise, is your greatest ally in maintaining a positive mental outlook, improving your overall health and well-being, and increasing your longevity and your quality of life.

What would happen if you were not active? This question is not difficult to answer. Most of us only have to look in the mirror. Gaining fat is a fairly slow process, and if we were to look carefully at our weight-loss dilemma in the rearview mirror, inactivity was the primary factor in getting to our present situation. How many years has it been since you graduated from school? If you gained 2 pounds every year since that date, would that be the weight you would now like to rid yourself of? The older we get, the less active we become. After we graduate from high school or college, we enter the workforce and become less active. When we become less active, we put on fat. We take on career responsibilities, spouse, and children, and have less time to spend on ourselves and less time engaged in physical activities. This has a significant psychological effect, and as we become fatter and less active, we become more prone to stress-related maladies like depression and anxiety. This causes an even more drastic reduction in our physical activity. After hitting middle age, we are much more likely to have heart disease, diabetes, and arthritis. This reduces our quality of life as we enter our golden years.

We can offset much of the aging process by even modest regular exercise. Some people recoil at the very word "exercise." Exercise is not a frightening concept. If you are not willing or able to train for a marathon, do not feel that you cannot do some kind of activity. Exercise is just an activity. The activity does not have to be strenuous. It can be as simple as walking. You burn as many calories by walking a mile as you do jogging a mile, you get the same heart and health benefits, and you are becoming active. The more active you are, the more activity you welcome into your daily life. It becomes a cycle. Instead of a decline in your physical activity, there is an increase. Instead of feeling anxiety, you have a new tool to combat stress. Instead of feelings of depression, increased activity promotes an entire realignment of the hormones that dictate mood and mental clarity, and you will feel uplifted, buoyant, and vital. As your physical activity increases, you become less fat and less susceptible to heart disease, diabetes, and arthritis. Look at Jack LaLanne. Exercise can offset the aging process and help you to be vital, self-sufficient, energized, and happy as you get older.

COMMITMENT TO LIFE

Begin increasing your activity by simply and realistically looking at your current activity level. Look at what you do every day. That is a great start. Could you do more of the things you are already doing? Have you always wanted to take on a certain sport or hobby? If you have always wanted to learn how to play tennis, here is your opportunity. Can you—more specifically, will you—do that? In addition to that new activity, is there something else you could do on the "off" days? Is there some kind of activity that you could do several times per week? Could you walk for 30 minutes a day? Would you walk for 30 minutes a day? Look at activity as something you could or would do for the rest of your life. The greatest thing you can do is to engage in regular activity. Just like brushing your teeth, this activity should be part of your daily routine. It is a commitment to yourself and to your future. The more active you are, the more active you become.

BENEFITS YOU CAN EXPECT TO RECEIVE FROM EXERCISE[11]

Feel Better

- Exercise alleviates depression by elevating the body's own naturally occurring painkilling substances called endorphins; these are the same substances thought to produce the "runner's high."
- According to a recent study, 90 percent of people surveyed say they feel better immediately after they exercise, and the effect is similar regardless of how long individuals have been exercising.
- Weight training has the same mood elevating effect as aerobic exercise.

Lose Weight

- A "balanced" diet is not enough to lose weight. Total calories, amount of fat, and fiber are key components of the diet plan.
- Exercise is equally important—many weight-loss programs fail because they are not built around a solid exercise program. To burn calories is essential—ultimately, that's how you lose the fat.
- Anyone can lose weight, but keeping it off is the challenge: weight loss is maintained with a lifelong nutrition and exercise program.

Improve Heart Health

- Cardiovascular disease continues to be the leading cause of death in America, claiming the lives of nearly one million individuals annually.
- An estimated one out of every four adults in the United States has high blood pressure.
- Regular aerobic exercise not only strengthens the heart but may even increase the size of the coronary blood vessels—reducing the risk of a heart attack.

ESTIMATED CREDITS PER HOUR OF EXERCISE[12]			
ACTIVITY	**IF YOU WEIGH**		
	100–150 POUNDS	**150–200 POUNDS**	**200 + POUNDS**
Archery	3	4	5
Backpacking (no load)	4	6	7
Backpacking (11-lb. load)	4	6	8
Backpacking (22-lb. load)	5	7	8
Backpacking (44-lb. load)	5	7	9
Badminton (recreation)	3	4	5
Badminton (competitive)	5	7	9
Baking	1	2	2
Baseball (player)	2	3	5
Baseball (pitcher)	3	4	6
Basketball (half court)	3	4	5
Basketball (moderate)	4	5	7
Basketball (competitive)	5	7	9
Bicycling (5.5 mph)	3	3	5
Bicycling (13 mph)	5	8	10
Bowling (nonstop)	3	3	3
Boxing (sparring)	3	4	5
Calisthenics	3	4	5
Canoeing (2.5 mph)	1	2	3
Canoeing (4 mph)	4	5	7
Car washing	2	3	4
Cardplaying	1	1	2

ACTIVITY	IF YOU WEIGH		
	100–150 POUNDS	150–200 POUNDS	200 + POUNDS
Carpentry	2	3	3
Carrying logs	6	9	11
Chopping (axe, slow)	3	4	6
Chopping (axe, fast)	10	14	18
Cleaning	2	3	4
Cooking	2	2	3
Cricket (batting)	3	4	5
Cricket (bowling)	3	4	5
Cricket (fielding)	3	4	5
Croquet	2	3	4
Dance, aerobic (easy)	3	5	6
Dance, aerobic (moderate)	4	5	6
Dance, aerobic (vigorous)	5	7	8
Dance, fox-trot	2	3	4
Dance, modern (vigorous)	3	4	6
Dance, rumba	4	5	7
Dance, square	3	5	7
Dance, waltz	3	4	5
Digging	5	7	9
Drawing (standing)	1	2	2
Driving (tractor)	1	2	2
Drum playing	2	3	4
Dusting	2	3	4
Fencing (moderate)	3	4	5
Fencing (competitive)	5	7	10
Field hockey	5	7	8
Fishing	2	3	4
Football (moderate)	3	4	5
Football (vigorous)	4	6	8
Frisbee	3	5	6
Golf (twosome)	3	4	5
Golf (foursome)	2	3	4

ACTIVITY	IF YOU WEIGH		
	100–150 POUNDS	150–200 POUNDS	200 + POUNDS
Handball	5	7	9
Hiking(40-lb. pack, 3 mph)	3	5	7
Hockey (ice)	5	8	9
Hoeing	3	4	5
Horseback riding (walk)	2	2	3
Horseback riding (trot)	3	5	7
Horseshoe pitching	2	3	3
Hunting	3	4	5
Ironing	1	2	2
Judo	6	9	12
Jumping rope (70/min)	6	8	10
Jumping rope (80/min)	6	8	10
Jumping rope (125/min)	6	9	10
Jumping rope (145/min)	7	10	12
Karate	6	9	12
Kendo	7	9	11
Knitting	1	1	1
Lacrosse	5	7	8
Marching (fast)	5	7	8
Mopping	2	3	4
Motorcycle riding	5	7	8
Mountain climbing	5	7	10
Mowing	4	5	7
Paddleball	5	7	9
Painting, inside	1	2	2
Painting, outside	3	4	5
Painting, scraping	2	3	4
Piano playing	1	2	2
Plastering	3	4	5
Pool, billiards	1	1	2
Raquetball	5	7	9
Raking	2	3	3

ACTIVITY	IF YOU WEIGH		
	100–150 POUNDS	150–200 POUNDS	200 + POUNDS
Roller skating	4	6	7
Running (11-min. mile)	5	8	10
Running (7-min. mile)	8	1	15
Running (5-min. mile)	10	14	19
Running (stationary, 140 counts/min)	12	17	23
Sprinting	12	17	22
Sailing	1	2	3
Sawing (power saw)	3	4	4
Sawing (by hand)	4	6	7
Scuba diving	7	9	10
Sewing (by hand)	1	1	1
Shopping for groceries	2	3	4
Sitting	1	1	1
Skateboarding	4	6	7
Skating (moderate)	3	4	6
Skating (vigorous)	5	7	10
Skiing (downhill)	5	7	9
Skiing (level, 5 mph)	8	12	16
Skin diving (moderate)	7	10	12
Skin diving (vigorous)	9	13	16
Snowmobiling	3	4	4
Soccer	5	6	9
Squash	5	7	10
Standing	1	1	2
Surfing	3	4	5
Swimming (recreational, 25 yds./min.)	3	4	6
Swimming (back, 20 yds./min.)	2	3	4
Swimming (back, 30 yds./min.)	3	4	5
Swimming (back, 40 yds./min.)	5	7	9
Swimming (butterfly, 50 yds./min.)	6	8	11
Swimming (crawl, 20 yds./min.)	2	3	5
Swimming (crawl, 45 yds./min.)	4	6	8

ACTIVITY	IF YOU WEIGH		
	100–150 POUNDS	150–200 POUNDS	200 + POUNDS
Swimming (crawl, 50 yds./min.)	5	8	10
Table tennis	2	3	4
Tennis (recreational)	3	5	7
Tennis (competitive)	5	7	9
Typing	1	1	2
Vacuuming	2	3	4
Volleyball (moderate)	3	4	6
Volleyball (vigorous)	5	7	9
Walking (2 mph)	2	3	3
Walking (110–120 steps/min.)	3	4	5
Washing (windows)	2	3	4
Washing (clothes)	2	3	4
Waterskiing	4	6	8
Weeding	2	4	4
Weight training	4	6	8
Welding	2	3	3
Wrestling	6	9	12
Writing	1	1	2

THE EQUATION IN ACTION

As you can clearly see, there are many ways that you can accumulate whatever credits you need. The more activities you can fit into your day, you will find yourself doing even more. Whether you choose to accumulate credits by reducing your caloric intake, or whether you choose to accumulate credits by increasing your activity level, or if you do a combination of both, it is important that you have some practical application to add all of these credits together.

By this time, you have gotten quite used to a daily worksheet or body bill. To bring all of this information into a practical application, it is essential that you continue to use the worksheet. This week you will add a layer to The Equation. These additions are credits and debits. You will see two columns with the heading "calories in" and "calories out." For each activity, you will fill in a credit. You have a choice in accounting for daily activities.

You may EITHER give yourself an automatic credit of three (3) for daily activities such as reading, writing, cooking, watching TV, etc., OR you can add all of these credits up using the "activities list" above; however, you MAY NOT add both. For any additional activity such as labor or exercise, consult the "activities list" and fill in the appropriate credit. Like last week, you will continue to account for each meal or snack, fill in what you ate, totaling up the debits. At the end of the day, you add up all of the "calories in." If it is exactly what you need, your total credits are zero; if it is more than what you need, you write in your total debits; if it is less than what you need, you are awarded 1 credit for every 100 calories. At the bottom of each worksheet you subtract the total debits from the total credits, and you are left with your total credits for the day.

The following example is of a 150-pound, 50-year-old woman with a fairly sedentary lifestyle. In determining what she could and would do to accumulate credits, this homemaker chose to reduce her caloric intake by 10 percent and commit to light physical activity each day by taking on the responsibility of walking the family dog. To reduce her caloric consumption, she studied what she was currently eating and tried to determine what she could part with. Her normal breakfast was a bagel with cream cheese, and coffee. She decided that she could eliminate the cream from her coffee and have just half of the bagel, and exchange regular cream cheese to a low-fat cream cheese. To her best estimation, this modest change would eliminate 150 calories or 10 percent of her ideal caloric intake.

BODY BILL EXAMPLE

DAY 1

Hour	Water	Meal	Foods	Calories/Debits	Total	Credits/Activity
1 wake up 7:00 Breakfast 7:35 **2** Snack 10:00	16 ounces WATER ✓	EAT ✓	1 tsp. cream cheese 1/2 bagel	50 100	150	1 Walked dog 30 min.
3					+	1 Baking (30 min.)
4 Lunch 12:30 **5**	16 ounces WATER ✓	EAT ✓	2 tsp. peanut butter 5 crackers celery	200 70 10	280	2 Played golf 1/2 Walked dog (15 min.)
6 Snack 3:00 **7** **8**	16 ounces WATER ✓	EAT ✓	lettuce mustard 4oz. chicken 2 sl. white bread	50 195 140	385	1 Vacuumed (30 min.) 1 Worked in garden (30 min.)
9 Dinner 6:00 **10** **11**	16 ounces WATER ✓	EAT ✓	2 tsp. peanut butter 1/2 cup cottage cheese 1oz. pretzels	23 120 110	253	1 Cooked dinner 1/2 Walked dog (15 min.)
12 **13** **14** **15** **16**		EAT ✓	1 cup salad 4 oz. fish 1/2 cup sweet potato	60 160 79	299	1 Walked dog (30 min.)

Subtract your ideal caloric intake	_1500_
from today's total caloric intake	− _1367_
	= _133_

IS THIS A CREDIT OR A DEBIT?

TOTAL DEBITS From Caloric Intake	Ø

TOTAL CREDITS From Caloric Reduction	→	1.33

TOTAL CREDITS
$10^1/_3$

TOTAL DEBITS	(−)	**TOTAL CREDITS**	(=)	**CREDITS FOR THE DAY** $10^1/_3$

ADJUSTING THE EQUATION

The Equation is flexible. When most people go off their "diet," they feel as if they failed, and they end up quitting. Not so with The Equation. If you overeat for one meal, or one day, you can always make up for the debit by accumulating more credits. If you mess up a meal, there are no Equation Police to knock on your door, and you shouldn't feel like a failure. Just recover from the setback as quickly as you can. Try to make up those debits by accumulating credits. Go for a long walk after dinner, play some tennis, play catch with the kids, do some kind of activity to make it up to yourself. You are accountable only to yourself.

DON'T TRY TO FOOL YOURSELF

The Equation works like clockwork. If you set a goal for yourself, and if you follow through every day, accumulating the number of credits you need to meet your weekly allotment, you will absolutely, positively meet that goal on time. If for some reason you do not, there is no scientific or physiological reason. If you are searching for such an answer, the best plan of action is to look closely at your meals. Did you account for *everything* that went in your mouth? Were there moments or periods where your eating became unconscious and you did not account for the debits? Without exception, you will meet your goals and get the results you desire if you follow the road map that is The Equation.

GETTING STARTED

We have provided seven days of worksheets. Before you fill them all in, we suggest that you make a copy for each day you plan to be using The Equation. You may want to place these worksheets in a binder and use them like a journal. We also suggest that you use these worksheets as a method to support your aspiration for a physical transformation and as a tool to meet your goals.

YOUR PERSONAL EQUATION

Before you begin, fill in the blanks.

Today I weigh _____ on the scale. If I add a zero on the end of my weight,

I know that I need _____ calories per day just to keep my heart beating

and my lungs breathing.

If you choose to reduce your caloric intake,
multiply your total calories by 10 percent.
For every 100 calories, you are awarded **1 credit**.

I can reduce my caloric intake by _____ calories per day.

At most, I can accumulate _____ credits by reducing my caloric intake.

I will accumulate _____ credits per day by increasing my level of activity.

Any activity that I do will count as a credit.

If I happen to take in more calories than I need to maintain my bodily func-

tions and the activity I engage in, it doesn't mean that I have failed. It

doesn't mean that I will quit. It just means that I will accumulate more cred-

its to meet my personal equation.

THE PROGRAM

1. This week you are tallying your calories in and subtracting that number from your ideal caloric intake.
2. You are examining your level of activity and equating that activity with a system of credits.
3. At the end of the day, you will use the body bill to add up credits and debits. For every 35 credits you accumulate, you will have lost 1 pound of fat.
4. To prevent your starvation-protection mechanism from becoming active, you can reduce your caloric intake by only 10 percent. Focus your attention on regular activity to accumulate the majority of your credits.
5. Begin to do regular activity each day. This is the last layer of your new lifestyle. Not only will regular activity and/or exercise dramatically affect your loss of fat, but it will also improve your health, your mental state, and your potential longevity.

WORKING THE EQUATION

1. Begin to layer in daily activity and exercise. Start by doing more of what you are already doing. Layer in a simple form of exercise, such as walking. Do this each day, make it part of your routine, and do it for the rest of your life.
2. To this new routine, you may decide to add more and more activity. The more active you are, the more active you will become. Try something you have always wanted to do. Take up a new hobby or a new sport.
3. If you exceed your ideal caloric intake, adjust the equation and offset overeating with additional activity.

WHAT YOU CAN EXPECT

The true variable in your transformation is your level of activity. If you are bedridden and reduce your ideal caloric intake by 10 percent you can expect to lose 1 pound every 2 to 3 weeks. If you are fairly sedentary, you may lose up to 1 pound every week. If you are moderately active, you might lose 1½ pounds every week. If you are extremely active, you will lose 2 pounds each and every week. Add those numbers up over 6 months or a year. Is this close to where you want to be?

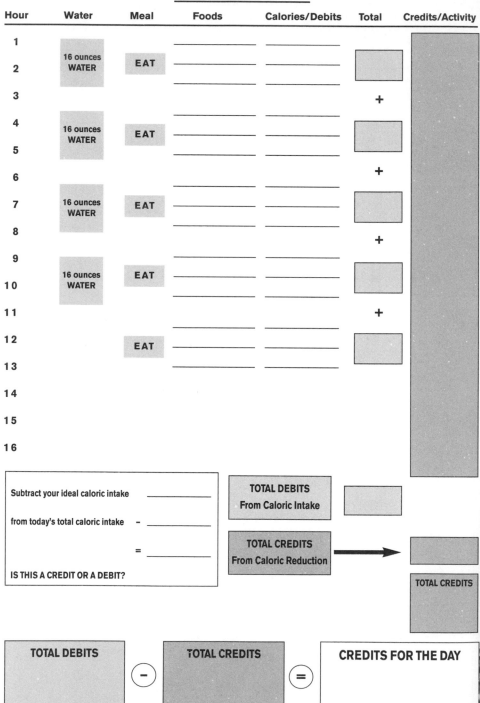

BODY BILL

DAY 2

Hour	Water	Meal	Foods	Calories/Debits	Total	Credits/Activity
1			_____	_____		
2	16 ounces WATER	EAT	_____	_____		
3			_____	_____	+	
4			_____	_____		
5	16 ounces WATER	EAT	_____	_____		
6			_____	_____	+	
7	16 ounces WATER	EAT	_____	_____		
8			_____	_____	+	
9			_____	_____		
10	16 ounces WATER	EAT	_____	_____		
11			_____	_____	+	
12		EAT	_____	_____		
13			_____	_____		
14						
15						
16						

Subtract your ideal caloric intake _____

from today's total caloric intake − _____

= _____

IS THIS A CREDIT OR A DEBIT?

TOTAL DEBITS
From Caloric Intake

TOTAL CREDITS
From Caloric Reduction ➔

TOTAL CREDITS

TOTAL DEBITS (−) **TOTAL CREDITS** (=) **CREDITS FOR THE DAY**

BODY BILL

DAY 3

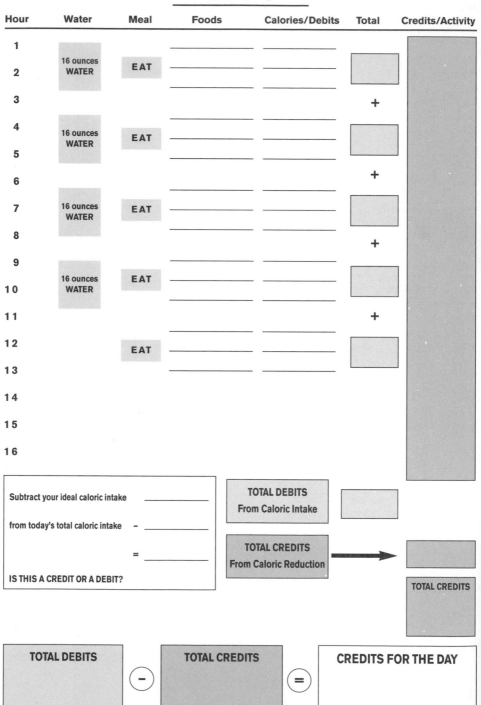

Hour	Water	Meal	Foods	Calories/Debits	Total	Credits/Activity
1						
2	16 ounces WATER	EAT				
3					+	
4	16 ounces WATER	EAT				
5						
6					+	
7	16 ounces WATER	EAT				
8					+	
9	16 ounces WATER	EAT				
10						
11					+	
12		EAT				
13						
14						
15						
16						

Subtract your ideal caloric intake _____

from today's total caloric intake − _____

= _____

IS THIS A CREDIT OR A DEBIT?

TOTAL DEBITS From Caloric Intake

TOTAL CREDITS From Caloric Reduction

TOTAL CREDITS

TOTAL DEBITS (−) **TOTAL CREDITS** (=) **CREDITS FOR THE DAY**

BODY BILL

DAY 4

Hour	Water	Meal	Foods	Calories/Debits	Total	Credits/Activity
1			_____	_____		
2	16 ounces WATER	EAT	_____	_____		
3			_____	_____	+	
4			_____	_____		
5	16 ounces WATER	EAT	_____	_____		
6			_____	_____	+	
7			_____	_____		
8	16 ounces WATER	EAT	_____	_____	+	
9			_____	_____		
10	16 ounces WATER	EAT	_____	_____		
11			_____	_____	+	
12		EAT	_____	_____		
13			_____	_____		
14						
15						
16						

Subtract your ideal caloric intake _____

from today's total caloric intake − _____

= _____

IS THIS A CREDIT OR A DEBIT?

TOTAL DEBITS
From Caloric Intake

TOTAL CREDITS
From Caloric Reduction ⟶

TOTAL CREDITS

TOTAL DEBITS	—	**TOTAL CREDITS**	=	**CREDITS FOR THE DAY**

BODY BILL

DAY 5

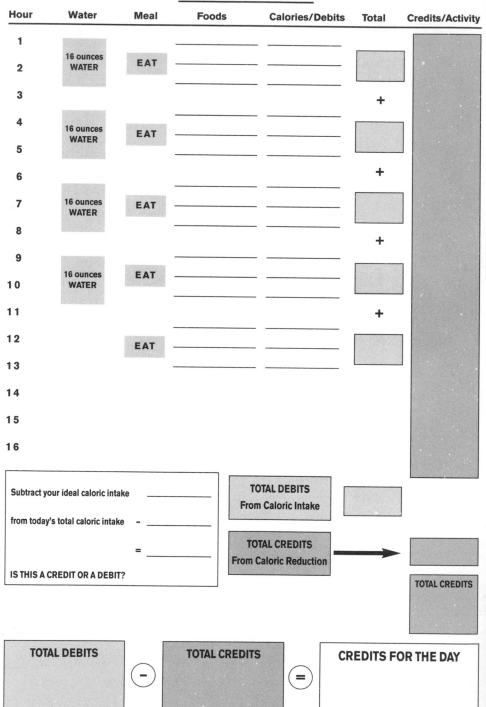

Hour	Water	Meal	Foods	Calories/Debits	Total	Credits/Activity
1						
2	16 ounces WATER	EAT				
3					+	
4						
5	16 ounces WATER	EAT				
6					+	
7	16 ounces WATER	EAT				
8					+	
9						
10	16 ounces WATER	EAT				
11					+	
12		EAT				
13						
14						
15						
16						

Subtract your ideal caloric intake _____

from today's total caloric intake − _____

= _____

IS THIS A CREDIT OR A DEBIT?

TOTAL DEBITS
From Caloric Intake

TOTAL CREDITS
From Caloric Reduction

TOTAL CREDITS

TOTAL DEBITS (−) **TOTAL CREDITS** (=) **CREDITS FOR THE DAY**

BODY BILL

DAY 6

Hour	Water	Meal	Foods	Calories/Debits	Total	Credits/Activity
1			_____	_____		
2	16 ounces WATER	EAT	_____	_____		
3			_____	_____	+	
4			_____	_____		
5	16 ounces WATER	EAT	_____	_____		
6			_____	_____	+	
7	16 ounces WATER	EAT	_____	_____		
8			_____	_____	+	
9			_____	_____		
10	16 ounces WATER	EAT	_____	_____		
11			_____	_____	+	
12		EAT	_____	_____		
13			_____	_____		
14						
15						
16						

Subtract your ideal caloric intake _____

from today's total caloric intake − _____

= _____

IS THIS A CREDIT OR A DEBIT?

TOTAL DEBITS
From Caloric Intake

TOTAL CREDITS
From Caloric Reduction

TOTAL CREDITS

TOTAL DEBITS	(−)	**TOTAL CREDITS**	(=)	**CREDITS FOR THE DAY**

BODY BILL

DAY 7

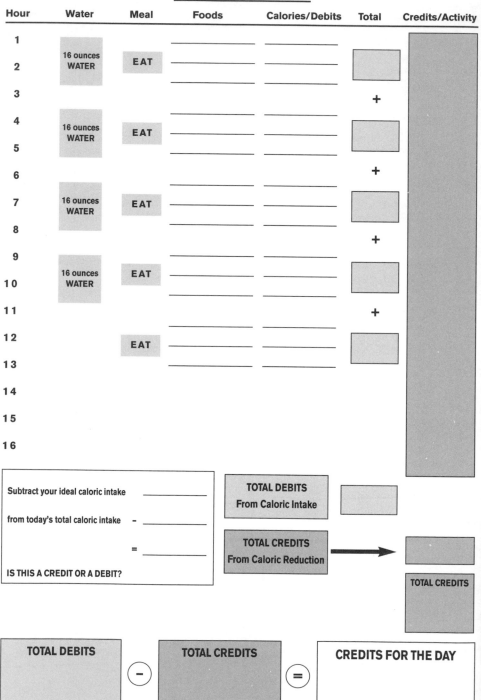

Hour	Water	Meal	Foods	Calories/Debits	Total	Credits/Activity
1						
2	16 ounces WATER	EAT				
3					+	
4						
5	16 ounces WATER	EAT				
6					+	
7	16 ounces WATER	EAT				
8					+	
9						
10	16 ounces WATER	EAT				
11					+	
12		EAT				
13						
14						
15						
16						

Subtract your ideal caloric intake _____

from today's total caloric intake − _____

= _____

IS THIS A CREDIT OR A DEBIT?

TOTAL DEBITS From Caloric Intake

TOTAL CREDITS From Caloric Reduction →

TOTAL CREDITS

TOTAL DEBITS (−) **TOTAL CREDITS** (=) **CREDITS FOR THE DAY**

CHAPTER EIGHT

Equation for Reaching Your Goal

In the first part of this book we stated that big change results can happen only by implementing small changes over time. In creating layer after layer of new habits you are developing a new lifestyle. These are precisely the small changes that will create a big change result. Your physical transformation is well under way, all the pieces are in place, and the only missing ingredients are time and a goal.

When you first began reading this book, we assume that you had a goal in mind. This chapter creates a context for the small changes you have made and will help you to apply what you are currently doing to meet a specific goal. Meeting your goal will take a strategy. There are two paths ahead of you. Which one you choose is completely dependent on your own personal needs, the time in which you want your big change results, and what you can and will do to get the results you desire.

To get the results you want you must have a goal in mind. Like anything else in life, setting a goal is a first step toward a big change result. After setting your goal, you will implement many small changes to reach that goal.

GOALS

The Equation is as simple as $1 + 1 = 2$, and "calories in" and "calories out" are the $1 + 1$. Now you need to figure out what happens after the $=$ sign. Last week, like every week, you filled out a body bill. At the end of each worksheet you arrived at a number. This number reflects and quantifies what you did for yourself in a 24-hour period. With that number, you have the key to reaching your goal. That is the key to your equation for results. The Equation can be adjusted, personalized, and customized to meet whatever goal you desire.

We are a goal-oriented society. We create goals for everything. We want to be married by a certain age. We want to save so much money before we have kids. We want to have so many children. We want to make so much money per year. We want to get such and such a return on that money when we invest it. We want to retire by a certain age. It goes on and on. In the context of losing fat, weight, and inches, you must create goals and find ways to achieve those goals each day.

It is essential that you create an overall goal for yourself. Even more essential is that your goal be realistic. Being realistic does not mean that you cannot shoot for the stars; it simply means that you should stay within the guidelines that we suggest as reasonable: Weight/fat loss over time is the best way to achieve results that last a lifetime. The most you can and should lose is about 2 pounds per week.

What is your ideal weight? If you could take your physical transformation to any level, where would that be, what would it look like, and what would you look like? This is called a long-term goal. Set this long-term goal as high as you want. You may want to lose 20, 50, or even 100 pounds. Now choose the date by which you will accomplish this goal. A successful strategy is to create a seasonal time line. If you begin this diet on January 1, set your goals by the season and work with dates that match. For instance, May 1, September 15, November 30, and March 15 are all dates that could mark the beginning of the seasons in your geographical location. You may consider losing so much in one year, or so much in two seasons, or so much in one season. During each season, you will have an objective to meet, and this will become a medium-term goal. You need to determine what you need to do each week to meet your medium-term goals. Then create a daily strategy to meet your weekly goals.

USING THE EQUATION TO MEET YOUR GOALS

What are your goals? How much do you want to lose? The table below shows how many credits you need to meet that goal. Along the left side are the number of pounds you would like to lose, and across the top is the number of weeks you need to meet those goals. Just like when you are trying to determine how many miles it is from one city to another, find where that number of weeks intersects with that number of pounds, and you will find the number of credits you need each week to meet that goal. Again, it is your objective to lose pounds of fat, not just random pounds, and the longer your fat loss takes, the more likely you will be to keep that fat off.

CREDITS PER WEEK REQUIRED TO LOSE DESIRED NUMBER OF FAT POUNDS IN DESIRED NUMBER OF WEEKS

LBS \ WKS	2	4	6	8	10	12	14	16	18	20	22	24	26	28	30	32	34	36	38	40	42	44	46	48	50	52
5		44	29	22	18	15	13	11	10	9	8	7	7	6	6	5	5	5	5	4	4	4	4	4	4	3
10			58	44	35	29	25	22	19	18	16	15	13	13	12	11	10	10	9	9	8	8	8	7	7	7
15				66	53	44	38	33	29	26	24	22	20	19	18	16	15	15	14	13	13	12	11	11	11	10
20					70	58	50	44	39	35	32	29	27	25	23	22	21	19	18	18	17	16	15	15	14	13
25							63	55	49	44	40	36	34	31	29	27	26	24	23	22	21	20	19	18	18	17
30								66	58	53	48	44	40	38	35	33	31	29	28	26	25	24	23	22	21	20
35									68	61	56	51	47	44	41	38	36	34	32	30	29	28	27	26	25	24
40										70	64	58	54	50	47	44	41	39	37	35	33	32	30	29	28	27
50													67	63	58	55	51	49	46	44	42	40	38	36	35	34
60															70	66	62	58	55	53	50	48	46	44	42	40
70																		68	64	61	58	56	53	51	49	47
80																				67	67	64	61	58	56	54
90																							68	66	63	61
100																								65	70	67

YOUR PERSONAL GOALS

You have determined that you want to lose _____ pounds of fat in _____ weeks. You used the table on the previous page and discovered that you need to accumulate _____ credits per week to meet that goal. Divide that number by 7 (the number of days in a week). Credits per week _____ ÷ 7 = _____ credits per day. To meet your goal, all you have to do is accumulate _____ credits per day. Because it has been tested over and over again, because The Equation is scientifically proven, because celebrities have used The Equation to get the results they desire, we can guarantee that if you accumulate _____ credits per week and _____ credits per day, if you continue to maintain the habits you have diligently created, you will absolutely, positively meet your goal. It is like clockwork.

How do you accumulate those credits? Again, there are only two strategies: reduce the number of calories you take in, and do more of the activities you are already doing or want to do. Let's get more specific and work it out here on paper. Let's really determine how you are going to get those credits, and what that would look like.

Your weight on the scale _____

Your weight on the scale + zero = _____

At rest, you need _____ calories per day just to maintain bodily functions.

It is safe to reduce that number by 10%.

Grand Total _____ × .10 = _____

For every 100 calories, you get 1 credit.

If you reduce your caloric intake by _____ calories you get _____ credits per day.

This number is significant. You can get a maximum of _____ credits per day by reducing your caloric intake. Accommodating this reduction is fairly simple. Refer to the food guide pyramid on page 62. All you have to do is continue accounting for each meal as you have been for the last few weeks.

Still, the problem is that you do not have enough credits each day just by reducing your caloric intake. You need _____ credits per day to meet your goal. By reducing your caloric intake you can win a maximum of _____ credits.

Daily credits to meet your goal _____–_____ credits from calorie reduction = _____. This is the number of calories you need to expend from additional activity.

Whatever activity you choose to do, there is a corresponding credit. The activity/exercise chart starting on page 104 tells you how many credits you can accumulate per hour. If you do 30 minutes of any given activity, divide the number in half. If you do 15 minutes, divide the number by 4, and so on.

Earlier, you created an entire series of goals. You created a long-term goal of how much fat, inches, and weight you want to lose. You set a date when you would like to realize those results. You then broke that time period down a bit more and discovered how many credits you need to accumulate each week, and how many credits you need each day to meet that goal. To follow through, you need to be able to apply all the information in The Equation. The Equation means nothing unless you can apply it to your life throughout the day. The greatest thing about The Equation is its flexibility. For instance, if you eat more than you should (debits), you can always cancel those debits out by doing more activities (credits). The main objective at the end of the day is to accumulate the number of credits you need to meet your daily goal.

Take a look at the following example. This 150-pound woman has a light activity level. It is her goal to lose 15 pounds in 12 weeks. By looking at the table, she discovered that she needs 44 credits per week, or 6.2 credits per day. She has decided to make a goal of earning 7 credits per day, with the hope that she will reach her goal even sooner.

This is the simple math she did before filling out the worksheet.

Her weight + a zero on the end = 1,500 calories.

She reduces her caloric intake by 10 percent. 1,500 × .10 = 150, or 1,350 calories per day.

She eats three meals and two snacks per day, so she decides that every time she eats, she will take in about 270 calories, for a total of 1,350 calories (a reduction of 150 calories).

She is awarded 1 credit for every 100 calories and discovers that she can get a total of 1½ credits just by reducing her caloric intake. Her goal is to earn 7 credits per day, so she needs to accumulate only 5½ credits per day through activity to reach her goal.

YOUR PERSONAL EQUATION

Before you begin, again fill in the blanks, so that you can restate your goals.

My goal is to lose _____ pounds by _____ / _____ / _____.

To achieve my goal, I will accumulate _____ credits per week.

To accumulate _____ credits per week, I will earn _____ credits per day.

Today I weigh _____ on the scale. If I add a zero on the end of my weight,

I know that I need _____ calories per day just to keep my heart beating

and my lungs breathing.

If you choose to reduce your caloric intake,
multiply your total calories by 10 percent.
For every 100 calories, you are awarded **1 credit**.

I can reduce my caloric intake by _____ calories per day.

At most, I can accumulate _____ credits by reducing my caloric intake.

To meet my goal, I will accumulate _____ credits per day by increasing

my level of activity.

Any activity that I do will count as a credit.

If I happen to take in more calories than I need to maintain my bodily func-

tions and the activity I engage in, it doesn't mean that I have failed. It

doesn't mean that I will quit. It just means that I will accumulate more cred-

its (refer to activity/exercise chart starting on page 104) to meet my per-

sonal equation.

WHAT THAT WOULD LOOK LIKE OVER TIME

If you accumulated that many credits per day, each day, what would that look like in a month? What would that look like in three months? What would that look like in nine months? It takes some vision to see this far into the future, but that is in fact a skill that you can develop easily.

If you were a movie star and were consulting with us, the last step of the consultation would be to put together a game plan for you. This game plan would come in the form of a calendar. On this calendar you would first write down your goal weight and the day you wanted to meet this goal. You would work backward from that date, creating several landmarks. Each week, you would have the total number of credits you need to accumulate to meet your goal, and each day you would write in the number of credits you actually accumulated. You can use your personal organizer or your wall calendar in a similar fashion.

THE PROGRAM

1. Set your long-term goal. Then set a medium-term goal. Then determine what you need to do each week to meet that goal.
2. Make copies of the body bill. Each day, accumulate the appropriate number of credits to meet your weekly goal.
3. Use a calendar to write in goal dates. Use this calendar by writing in how many *credits* you earned each day.
4. Be accountable for meeting your goal.

You now have all the tools you need. You have all the information you need. All that is left is to work your own equation each day. Accumulate a specific number of credits each day. Stay on track to meet your weekly goals, and in no time at all you will have achieved your goal. You have the road map, just follow it. If you get detoured, read the chapter in part four that is most appropriate for your goal weight for some additional suggestions. When you have reached your goal, read the last chapter on maintenance.

CUSTOMIZING

The

EQUATION

This section of the book is devoted to goal-oriented achievement. In truth, you have developed all the tools you need to complete your physical transformation, and there is little else to say, or suggest, or demonstrate. All that is left is to provide you with the context to apply your new lifestyle habits toward your own personal goal.

The goal that you create for yourself is profound. It represents much more than to "lose a few pounds." Your goal represents your aspirations for a better life, a life with a higher quality. Thus far, you have put in the time and effort to create a change in your life, and by layering in several small patterns of behavior, we hope that this has helped you in creating quality to some degree. Realistically, you should be noticing a difference in your energy level—you should notice that your higher energy level does not have peaks and valleys during the day but stays even throughout. You should feel more focused, more clearheaded. You may sense that you are more in touch with your body than you were a few weeks back. You may notice that your digestive process and almost all of your bodily functions are operating more efficiently. You may be enjoying what you eat more than ever before. You may even have had a profound experience while sharing quality time and quality eating with friends and family. You should be noticing that you are more active, and this should have many benefits such as feelings of well-being, reduced stress, and vitality. In short, The Equation offers many benefits that can be enjoyed throughout your day. Those are the things you get as a result of what you are doing. Truly, these are the results you are looking for. In addition, you may also have to purchase a new wardrobe.

When most of us think about results, we think in terms of the bottom line. In terms of physical transformation, you probably think of results in terms of pounds, or inches, or clothes sizes. Without doubt, you are on the road to achieving those results, and to get there you only need a road map. This section of the book is dedicated to helping you to set reasonable goals and personalizing The Equation to meet those goals.

CHAPTER NINE

The Equation for Losing 5 Pounds

If you are looking to lose 5 pounds in the next two weeks, there is much good news. The best news is that the lifestyle habits that allowed you to gain the extra 5 pounds can be easily reversed. Losing those 5, or even 20 pounds, is really and truly a function of your lifestyle. If, for some reason, you have opened up the book and are just beginning at this point, we caution you to stop and start at the beginning.

If you have read this book from the beginning and have been following our suggestions for these last weeks, you should be well on your way toward meeting your goal. Perhaps you have already lost some weight on the scale and would like to lose an additional 5 pounds of fat. In either case, we provide some suggestions to help you reach your goal.

If you have been following each step in this book, you have made many positive and beneficial adjustments in your lifestyle to accommodate a shift in the way your particular body rids itself of fat. With some small adjustments, you should have no problem reaching your goal. As always, there are three ways to create a strategy to reach this goal.

1. You can merely reduce the number of calories you are eating and reach your goal. Because you can reduce your caloric intake by 10 percent, it will take a few weeks to reach your destination, but you will get there.

2. You can accumulate the credits you need by just increasing your activity level. This is quite simple. You could continue to eat five appropriately portioned meals but walk two miles (30 minutes) each day.

3. You can reduce your caloric intake by 10 percent *and* increase your level of activity.

As always, it is our suggestion that you do both, as this creates the ideal environment to foster fat loss, and it ensures that you receive all the mental and health benefits of regular exercise.

OBSTACLES

We are all different individuals, with differing needs and circumstances. All of us face challenges. There are obstacles that exist for you, and you should see them as factors that will challenge your will and desire. Obstacles and challenges can and will be overcome, but it is essential that they are at least acknowledged. There are three primary factors and three potential obstacles that all of us need to address: age, stress level, and time. You need to realize that your age, your stress level, and your time have all been factors in putting on the weight you now want to lose. When we speak of lifestyle, and making adjustments, we are really talking about how to affect these three critical areas.

Our level of stress and our time are directly linked to the number of responsibilities we have. The older we get, the more responsibilities we take on. It is quite possible that when you graduated from school you were much leaner than you are today. In those days, you had plenty of time for recreation. When you began a career or got married, that recreational time for activity was reduced. As you advanced in your work and/or had children, that recreational time spent on activity was diminished even further. The bottom line is that we all have responsibilities, and very often our last priority is ourselves. We would like to reiterate a simple profound truth: Your time is your own until you give it away. You can, in fact, reduce your level of stress by becoming more active. Even if it is a 15-minute walk, you will feel far less uptight when you are finished. Time is what you need to create. If you look carefully at your daily schedule, no matter how hectic or frenetic your pace, we guarantee you can find an hour in your day. This hour may typically be spent "relaxing." It may be an hour you typically watch television. It may be the hour you spend drinking coffee or reading the paper. It may be 10 minutes here and 30 minutes there, but somehow or other you can squeeze in an hour to fulfill your goal.

When you do find this hour, don't think of it as "selfish" time. Take a walk with your spouse. Play with the kids or grandchildren. Spend that time doing helpful projects to improve your home or yard. Spend the time doing something you enjoy. Have fun. You deserve joy, and if you look at your activity as "having fun," chances are you will do more of it. If you can find some room in your life for a little bit more joy, you will have more to pass around to those you love. This time will be spent improving your life, and as a result, the quality of life of those you touch will be improved as well.

SUBSTITUTE, MODIFY, AND SHIFT

As always, the name of the game is staying on the plan. Staying on the plan does not mean that if you happen to fall, you cannot recover and get back on your feet. The Equation is relatively forgiving in that if you make a mistake there are many opportunities to make up for it. Still, at all times try to stay the course. There will be challenges and obstacles, but to a large degree there are three ways to effectively overcome those hurdles.

To reach your goal and lose an additional 5 pounds, you will have to adhere to the basic principle of The Equation. Meeting your goal is all about calories in and calories out. You will have to do everything in your power to make the commitment to create your own personal strategy and stick to it. If you are looking to adhere to your strategy and face obstacles that need to be overcome, your best options are to modify, substitute, or shift.

YOUR STRATEGY TO LOSE 5 POUNDS

It is unusual if you have not achieved your goal by following the suggestions in Chapters 2 through 5. However, by your diligent attention to these directions, you have narrowed considerably the possible causes for your condition. The bottom line is that you will not have a problem achieving your goal of losing 5 pounds. You are very close to your goal. You need only minor lifestyle adjustments to reach it.

Losing 5 pounds takes very little effort, and it is a goal that you can easily achieve. Many celebrities fall into this category. (In fact, most of us fall into this category at one time or another, especially after the holidays.) Actors are hired for a film that begins shooting in two weeks, and they have to get in the best shape possible for when they get in front of the camera.

There are two ways you can adjust The Equation to meet your goal. The first course of action is to increase your level of activity or do the activities you are already doing for a longer time. The second course of action is to take a close look at what you are putting into your mouth. Chances are that you are overeating or eating the wrong foods. The primary nutritional changes we suggest are to be certain you are not eating too much food at any given meal. Again, the object of the exercise is to eat several small meals spaced throughout the day, and eat every 2½ to 3 hours or so. If you are already doing this religiously, there are two other places to look. The major culprit could very well be the amount of fat you are eating. All foods have traces of fat, and fat definitely does give food a fuller flavor, but for the next two weeks, we want you to use only the fat that you cook your food in. Eliminate all fast food and all deep-fried foods during this 14-day period. When possible, use cooking spray to coat the pan instead of using butter or oil. Lastly, eat less beef, lamb, and pork, and replace those protein choices with skinless chicken or turkey breast, fish, seafood, or soy products.

GETTING SPECIFIC

Achieving your goal requires you to be specific about the total calories you are eating each day, and about the total calories you are burning off each day. To achieve your goal you have to burn off more calories than you take in. Just as in the last chapter, getting specific means that you use The Equation to burn off the number of calories needed to achieve your goal. Your goal is to lose 5 pounds. To achieve your goal, you need to focus in on what you will do each day to achieve your goal. To lose 5 pounds, you have to accumulate a total of 175 credits.

At most, you should accumulate 70 credits per week, which comes out to about 10 credits per day. Although you could lose this "weight" at a faster pace, the goal is to lose *fat* and keep it off. Therefore, at the most rapid and safest pace, meeting your goal will take you about 18 days.

Here is an example of a calendar that reflects your exact goal. You should create one of these for yourself and use it each day. By making the appropriate number of body bills, you can also get really specific about what you are doing each day to meet your goal.

EQUATION CREDIT CALENDAR

DAY 1	DAY 2	DAY 3	DAY 4	DAY 5	DAY 6	DAY 7
1 Calories in–3 Calories out–2 Total–5	2 Calories in–3 Calories out–2 Total–5	3 Calories in–3 Calories out–2 Total–5	4 Calories in–3 Calories out–3 Total–6	5 Calories in–3 Calories out–3 Total–6	6 Calories in–3 Calories out–3 Total–6	7 Calories in–3 Calories out–3 Total–6 Total Week–39
8 Calories in–3 Calories out–2 Total–5	9 Calories in–3 Calories out–2 Total–5	10 Calories in–3 Calories out–2 Total–5	11 Calories in–3 Calories out–3 Total–6	12 Calories in–3 Calories out–3 Total–6	13 Calories in–3 Calories out–3 Total–6	14 Calories in–3 Calories out–3 Total–6 Total Week–39
15 Calories in–3 Calories out–2 Total–5	16 Calories in–3 Calories out–2 Total–5	17 Calories in–3 Calories out–2 Total–5	18 Calories in–3 Calories out–3 Total–6	19 Calories in–3 Calories out–3 Total–6	20 Calories in–3 Calories out–3 Total–6	21 Calories in–3 Calories out–3 Total–6 Total Week–39
22 Calories in–3 Calories out–2 Total–5	23 Calories in–3 Calories out–2 Total–5	24 Calories in–3 Calories out–3 Total–6	25 Calories in–3 Calories out–3 Total–6	26 Calories in–3 Calories out–3 Total–6	27 Calories in–3 Calories out–3 Total–6	28 Calories in–3 Calories out–3 Total–6 Total Week–40
29 Calories in–3 Calories out–3 Total–6	30 Calories in–3 Calories out–3 Total–6	31 Calories in–3 Calories out–3 Total–6 Total Week–18				Total Month–175 Total Fat Loss– 5 pounds

EQUATION CREDIT CALENDAR

DAY 1	DAY 2	DAY 3	DAY 4	DAY 5	DAY 6	DAY 7
1 Calories in– Calories out– Total–	2 Calories in– Calories out– Total–	3 Calories in– Calories out– Total–	4 Calories in– Calories out– Total–	5 Calories in– Calories out– Total–	6 Calories in– Calories out– Total–	7 Calories in– Calories out– Total– Total Week–
8 Calories in– Calories out– Total–	9 Calories in– Calories out– Total–	10 Calories in– Calories out– Total–	11 Calories in– Calories out– Total–	12 Calories in– Calories out– Total–	13 Calories in– Calories out– Total–	14 Calories in– Calories out– Total– Total Week–
15 Calories in– Calories out– Total–	16 Calories in– Calories out– Total–	17 Calories in– Calories out– Total–	18 Calories in– Calories out– Total–	19 Calories in– Calories out– Total–	20 Calories in– Calories out– Total–	21 Calories in– Calories out– Total– Total Week–
22 Calories in– Calories out– Total–	23 Calories in– Calories out– Total–	24 Calories in– Calories out– Total–	25 Calories in– Calories out– Total–	26 Calories in– Calories out– Total–	27 Calories in– Calories out– Total–	28 Calories in– Calories out– Total– Total Week–
29 Calories in– Calories out– Total–	30 Calories in– Calories out– Total–	31 Calories in– Calories out– Total– Total Week–			Total Month–	Total Fat Loss– — pounds

CHAPTER TEN

The Equation for Losing 20 Pounds

If you want to lose 20 pounds the news is still good. The reason you have put on those 20 "extra" pounds is that your lifestyle choices have led you to this point. Like the person who wants to lose 5 pounds, these lifestyle habits are the main factor in your weight gain, but these habits have just been going on for a longer period of time. Just like the person who wants to lose 5 pounds, adjusting your lifestyle will facilitate your goal with little or no problem.

The issue here is really creeping obesity. It is an issue that we discussed earlier in the book, but it deserves to be repeated here. One morning you wake up and say, "Where did this spare tire come from?" It didn't arrive in your sleep. It accumulated over time, and it will take some time to be rid of it. Without even realizing that it is happening, you may gain a pound or two every year. So when you are 60, you are 40 to 80 pounds heavier than you were when you were 20. You need to become more accountable to yourself in terms of the amount of time you are allowing for the most important person in your life—you.

YOUR STRATEGY TO LOSE 20 POUNDS

If you are looking to lose twenty pounds, your age is certainly a factor in how that "extra" weight came to be. Take a look at your life over the last five or ten years. Has your activity level slowed down at all? Whether you are 18 or 80, you can be more active than you are today. This does not mean that you need to be in training for a marathon, it just means that the more active you are, the younger you will feel at any age.

When you have 20 pounds of body fat that you would like to lose, you have some unique needs and concerns. In large part that extra weight has been put on as a result of lifestyle choices. In almost all cases, these lifestyle issues revolve around age and responsibilities. Essentially, you have either become less active because of your age, or the responsibilities you have taken on preclude you from regular exercise. If this rings true for you, it is essential that you understand the imbalance that is present in your life that has caused the condition you would like to reverse.

I have trained many celebrities who fall within this category. Usually the actors who come to me wanting to lose 20 pounds don't necessarily need to, but rather they have to lose that amount of weight to be better suited for a role. For anyone who wants to lose 20 pounds, it is important to add more activity—especially aerobic activity. For Robin Williams, it was all about finding a form of exercise he was passionate about. Today he is cycling and even competes on a very high level. For all of them, the secret was in discovering what they could feel passionate about, and focusing on what they enjoyed. The same will hold true for you.

On this particular diet plan, the area that you are going to focus most on is exercise. The problem may lie in the fact that you either need to increase the duration of your exercise, or find a new form of exercise that burns more calories or gets a more beneficial response from your body. If your age is affecting your activity level, there are many low-impact and non-impact activities to participate in. Activity begets activity, and this means just getting started and finding something you are comfortable doing. Do you exercise now?

If you do not exercise because of other responsibilities, the answer lies in your schedule. For you, the biggest consideration is time. We all have commitments and responsibilities, so it is essential to create some time each day to fit in some kind of structured exercise. It doesn't matter if it is just 30 minutes, you need to give yourself that time. Perhaps you can ride a bicycle to work. Perhaps you can jog or play basketball at the Y during lunchtime. If you have a lunch meeting, schedule it within a mile of your office and walk back and forth. There is usually some time in your day that you have reserved to "relax." Perhaps you tune out in front of the television after dinner. Take a walk instead. Chances are you will actually be more relaxed and have a clearer head after a 30-minute walk than if you watched three hours of television. If you just cannot do without your TV fix, perhaps you can get a treadmill, stair climber, or exercise bike and exercise while you take in your favorite shows. If you have time to take up a new hobby, make it something that requires you to be active. Perhaps you would like to play golf or tennis or join a softball league. Maybe you live near the water and always wanted to surf, kayak, or row a racing scull. Perhaps you live in a climate where winter is severe. You could learn to play squash, cross-country ski, figure skate, or swing dance. Perhaps you have always wanted to hire a trainer and really learn how to work out. Go for it! Find something you like to do. Try something you always wanted to do. Get active! The more active you are, you will find that you become even more active. It becomes a cycle that grows and grows, gaining momentum by the amount of activity you can squeeze in each day.

For the first week, make a commitment to get in at least 30 minutes of activity each day. In the second week, increase that time to 45 minutes. In the third week, increase your activity time to 55 minutes. The fourth week, get in one hour per day. Finding the time to accommodate an hour might seem overwhelming to you right now, but really reflect on how your day is spent. Could you find 30 minutes to walk back and forth to lunch? Could you spend 30 minutes taking a walk with your spouse or children? Could you schedule a meeting playing golf or tennis instead of in a conference room? Could you get up 30 minutes earlier and jump rope? Could you walk the stairs at your office a few times before or after lunch? However busy you are, you can find the time. This time is for yourself, and for your future. If you are so busy that you cannot find 30 extra minutes, you truly *need* to find a release for the stress of that heavy workload.

To remain accountable to yourself for meeting your goal, we strongly suggest that you use a body bill each day and be ultraconscious of accumulating activity credits. Then create a calendar to reach your goal. The safest and quickest time frame you could reach your goal is 10 weeks from today. If this seems too far in the future for your personal taste, please consider the fact that you will enjoy many benefits each and every day during this time. In a relatively short period of time (just one season of the year), you will look and feel much different than you do today.

The following calendars represent how your transformation might look if you wanted to lose 8 pounds per month (20 pounds in 10 weeks) or 5 pounds per month (20 pounds in four months). You could choose to take more time to lose the same amount, and decide that losing 20 pounds in 12 months fits more appropriately into your life. The following calendars are just a visual aid to show you how easy losing 20 pounds of fat can be.

EQUATION CREDIT CALENDAR

DAY 1	DAY 2	DAY 3	DAY 4	DAY 5	DAY 6	DAY 7
1 Calories in–3 Calories out–2 Total–5	2 Calories in–3 Calories out–2 Total–5	3 Calories in–3 Calories out–2 Total–5	4 Calories in–3 Calories out–3 Total–6	5 Calories in–3 Calories out–3 Total–6	6 Calories in–3 Calories out–3 Total–6	7 Calories in–3 Calories out–3 Total–6 Total Week–39
8 Calories in–3 Calories out–2 Total–5	9 Calories in–3 Calories out–2 Total–5	10 Calories in–3 Calories out–2 Total–5	11 Calories in–3 Calories out–3 Total–6	12 Calories in–3 Calories out–3 Total–6	13 Calories in–3 Calories out–3 Total–6	14 Calories in–3 Calories out–3 Total–6 Total Week–39
15 Calories in–3 Calories out–2 Total–5	16 Calories in–3 Calories out–2 Total–5	17 Calories in–3 Calories out–2 Total–5	18 Calories in–3 Calories out–3 Total–6	19 Calories in–3 Calories out–3 Total–6	20 Calories in–3 Calories out–3 Total–6	21 Calories in–3 Calories out–3 Total–6 Total Week–39
22 Calories in–3 Calories out–2 Total–5	23 Calories in–3 Calories out–2 Total–5	24 Calories in–3 Calories out–3 Total–6	25 Calories in–3 Calories out–3 Total–6	26 Calories in–3 Calories out–3 Total–6	27 Calories in–3 Calories out–3 Total–6	28 Calories in–3 Calories out–3 Total–6 Total Week–40
29 Calories in–3 Calories out–3 Total–6	30 Calories in–3 Calories out–3 Total–6	31 Calories in–3 Calories out–3 Total–6 Total Week–18				Total Month–175 Total Fat Loss– 5 pounds

EQUATION CREDIT CALENDAR

DAY 1	DAY 2	DAY 3	DAY 4	DAY 5	DAY 6	DAY 7
1 Calories in–4 Calories out–5 Total–9	2 Calories in–4 Calories out–5 Total–9	3 Calories in–4 Calories out–5 Total–9	4 Calories in–4 Calories out–5 Total–9	5 Calories in–4 Calories out–5 Total–9	6 Calories in–4 Calories out–5 Total–9	7 Calories in–4 Calories out–5 Total–9 Total Week–63
8 Calories in–4 Calories out–5 Total–9	9 Calories in–4 Calories out–5 Total–9	10 Calories in–4 Calories out–5 Total–9	11 Calories in–4 Calories out–5 Total–9	12 Calories in–4 Calories out–5 Total–9	13 Calories in–4 Calories out–5 Total–9	14 Calories in–4 Calories out–5 Total–9 Total Week–63
15 Calories in–4 Calories out–5 Total–9	16 Calories in–4 Calories out–5 Total–9	17 Calories in–4 Calories out–5 Total–9	18 Calories ir–4 Calories out–5 Total–9	19 Calories in–4 Calories out–5 Total–9	20 Calories in–4 Calories out–5 Total–9	21 Calories in–4 Calories out–5 Total–9 Total Week–63
22 Calories in–4 Calories out–5 Total–9	23 Calories in–4 Calories out–5 Total–9	24 Calories in–4 Calories out–5 Total–9	25 Calories in–4 Calories cut–5 Total–9	26 Calories in–4 Calories out–5 Total–9	27 Calories in–4 Calories out–5 Total–9	28 Calories in–4 Calories out–5 Total–9 Total Week–63
29 Calories in–4 Calories out–5 Total–9	30 Calories in–4 Calories out–5 Total–9	31 Calories in–4 Calories out–5 Total–9 Total Week–27			Total Month–279	Total Fat Loss– 8 pounds

EQUATION CREDIT CALENDAR

DAY 1	DAY 2	DAY 3	DAY 4	DAY 5	DAY 6	DAY 7
1 Calories in– Calories out– Total–	2 Calories in– Calories out– Total–	3 Calories in– Calories out– Total–	4 Calories in– Calories out– Total–	5 Calories in– Calories out– Total–	6 Calories in– Calories out– Total–	7 Calories in– Calories out– Total– Total Week–
8 Calories in– Calories out– Total–	9 Calories in– Calories out– Total–	10 Calories in– Calories out– Total–	11 Calories in– Calories out– Total–	12 Calories in– Calories out– Total–	13 Calories in– Calories out– Total–	14 Calories in– Calories out– Total– Total Week–
15 Calories in– Calories out– Total–	16 Calories in– Calories out– Total–	17 Calories in– Calories out– Total–	18 Calories in– Calories out– Total–	19 Calories in– Calories out– Total–	20 Calories in– Calories out– Total–	21 Calories in– Calories out– Total– Total Week–
22 Calories in– Calories out– Total–	23 Calories in– Calories out– Total–	24 Calories in– Calories out– Total–	25 Calories in– Calories out– Total–	26 Calories in– Calories out– Total–	27 Calories in– Calories out– Total–	28 Calories in– Calories out– Total– Total Week–
29 Calories in– Calories out– Total–	30 Calories in– Calories out– Total–	31 Calories in– Calories out– Total– Total Week–				Total Month– Total Fat Loss– __ pounds

CHAPTER ELEVEN

The Equation for Losing 50 Pounds or More

Losing 50 or 100 pounds *can* be done, and you can and will do it. If you are reading these words, you obviously think you have that much weight to lose, and there are many reasons why you should. The object of this exercise is not for you to look like a supermodel. The object of this exercise is to improve your prospects for a healthy, long life.

More than any other reader, this book has been written for you. This book is not structured as a quick fix. You cannot possibly lose the weight you want to lose overnight, and you shouldn't be approaching any nutritional program or other medical option as a total answer. The fact of the matter is that in your present condition your long-term health is being compromised. If you can alter your course at this point, much of these health issues can and will be reversed. The time to alter your life is now. We want to lend a hand.

If you want to lose more than 50 pounds, there are some issues that need to be addressed. First, you need to congratulate yourself for even picking up this book. It needs to be acknowledged that you are a courageous person. Being overweight in this society is not what most of us consider a joyride. From shopping to advertising to the depiction of heavy people in movies and television, being overweight is truly challenging to one's psyche. You have not resigned yourself, you have not given up, you have not lost hope, and you are fighting to change your body, your appearance, and your life. For this, and this alone, you should hold your head high. You are spirited and brave. You should feel very proud. We have written this book and this chapter specifically as a tool for your ultimate victory.

Whether you were a heavy child and were teased, whether you were traumatized by the "husky" section of your clothing store as an adolescent, whether you feel like you missed out on romantic or job opportunities, or whether being overweight precludes you from participating in activities with others, being overweight makes you feel "different" and apart. There is significant emotional baggage that comes with being overweight, and this might be an appropriate time to begin sorting out that baggage. Much of this chapter is devoted to your emotional orientation to being overweight and to the way you are currently eating. Before we wade into these issues, it is appropriate to look at how your present condition came to be.

CAUSATIVE FACTORS

There are many reasons why this condition might be present and many possible answers why you are carrying more weight than you would like. There could be a medical explanation for why you are overweight. There could be a psychological reason. Your extra weight could be due to a hereditary predisposition. Your weight gain could be an emotional or chemical reaction to the food you are eating. Your weight may be attributed to an emotional response to food. All or many of these factors may have a cluster effect on your present condition. We can point the way toward possibilities, but we cannot create the solution. While we discuss these factors below, we can only help to point the way toward solutions for them. It is up to you to seek the proper professional guidance, but once you do, the remainder of this chapter will still serve as the strategy to meet your goal.

MEDICAL EXPLANATIONS

The human body is a vast and complex system of organs and hormones. There are organs that regulate the amount of fat we carry around and other organs that regulate the way fats, glucose, and proteins are placed within our fat cells. The primary organ responsible for regulating the fat we put on, otherwise known as our metabolism, is generally referred to as the endocrine system and specifically referred to as our thyroid gland. If you have 50 or more pounds to lose, we suggest that you at least rule out a thyroid gland malfunction by seeing a medical professional. A wide range of problems can affect the thyroid, either causing it to become underactive (hypothyroidism) or overactive (hyperthyroidism). Often, the symptoms of these conditions can be interchanged. In other words, you may have some classic symptoms of hypothyroidism and other symptoms of classic hyperthyroidism. Look over these classic symptoms, and if many of the symptoms from either condition apply to you, it may warrant a consultation with your doctor or even a specialist.

HYPOTHYROIDISM	HYPERTHYROIDISM
• slow heartbeat	• accelerated heartbeat
• fatigue	• weak and shaky muscles
• intolerance to cold	• excess sweating
• slower mental processes	• intolerance to hot weather
• poor memory	• weight loss
• weight gain	• restlessness
• constipation	• anxiety
• dry, brittle skin, nails, and hair	• insomnia
• elevated cholesterol	• frequent bowel movements
• swollen ankles and puffiness around the face	• eye problems
• goiter (enlargement of the thyroid gland)	• goiter

PSYCHOLOGICAL FACTORS

Many people who are 50 pounds overweight have encountered some degree of psychological trauma. If you could look at life through the rearview mirror and trace your personal history back to a time when you weren't heavy, there may have been some event that triggered your weight gain. Without getting into the realm of pop psychology, this trauma or traumatic event still may be just below the surface. When such an event has occurred, the weight we tend to put on acts as a barrier to protect ourselves from more emotional pain. Seen in the context of some kind of emotional armor, the weight you would now like to rid yourself of has been part of a defense mechanism. In other words, ridding yourself of this extra weight may be more difficult than lowering your caloric intake or increasing your level of activity. On a psychological, spiritual, or emotional level, there may be some deep-seated subconscious need for you to have this barrier, this armor. Your conscious mind knows that this extra weight cannot protect you from being hurt. You know that, if anything, this extra weight has been the specific source of much pain. However, our subconscious is quite strong and persuasive. If your conscious mind can say one thing, and your subconscious is working against you, it can only lead to conflict. Often this conflict results in truly negative thoughts that center upon our self-worth. Any words of encouragement, any words of advice will be just that—only words. There are many places you can look for answers. Certainly, professional counselors or therapists are a logical place to find support. However difficult the journey of healing these issues may be, there will be an amazingly rich payoff.

PREDISPOSITION TO OBESITY

Genetic predisposition can play a role in your current situation. Most of us were not destined to look like a stick-figure drawing. Most of us need only to look at our parents or our grandparents to understand what was inherited. Like any gene that is passed down, all of us are born with a certain number of inherited fat cells. What we do with those fat cells is within our control. As we stated earlier, any fat cell can shrink to an almost microscopic size, or can grow to the size of a grapefruit or cantaloupe.

CHEMICAL REACTION AND/OR DEPENDENCE ON FOOD

Much like alcohol or drug dependency, most of us who have 50 or 100 pounds to lose also have a food addiction. During the 1980s "chemical dependency" became an official disease that had prescribed and proven methods of treatment. When broken down to the most basic molecular level, the food you eat is made up of many different chemical compounds. Some of us eat compulsively or unconsciously. Some of us eat to provide comfort. Some of us eat to offset stress. When alcoholics or smokers are faced with an uncomfortable or stressful situation, their conscious or unconscious response is to take a drink or light up. In doing so, they are altering the chemicals in their body. Chances are that you are doing the same thing with food. Have you ever seen children eat a great quantity of candy? They get all hopped up on sugar, and it changes their personality a little bit. They might be a little wild, they might not listen as closely, or they might misbehave a little, and because of the change in their behavior, you notice. You may be having the same kind of response to the food you eat. Things might get stressful at work and you reach for something to eat. The cliché that when a breakup occurs, ice cream and chocolate soon follow is not too far from the truth. More often than not, when we eat to alter our chemical makeup, we reach for something sweet or a simple carbohydrate like bread or pasta. Just like kids on Halloween night, that sweet or carbo-hydrate sends a chemical through our bloodstream and into our brain. Just like the smoker, the drug addict, or the alcoholic, we get relief from the food we eat. While an alcoholic can quit drinking, while a drug addict can quit doing drugs, while a smoker can stop smoking, you cannot stop eating. You need to eat to live. However, there is a pattern of behavior that you can break, and that is the behavior of eating unconsciously or out of emotional need. Following The Equation and filling in the daily worksheet will do much to help you break this pattern of behavior.

There are specific times when you will be required to eat, and specific guidelines for what and how much you should eat. From this moment forward, you will be accountable for what you put into your mouth. If you notice that you are eating at a time when it is not prescribed, or if you notice that you are eating a greater quantity than is prescribed, you need to make some notes. For every day that you follow The Equation, until you meet your goal, you must fill in a daily worksheet. Using this worksheet will help you to keep track of your progress each day. In addition to using this worksheet like a daily journal, we highly recommend that you make copies of the following pages and place them in the back of your journal. When you find yourself eating at an unspecified time, or going beyond the boundaries of the suggested portion size, simply fill in the blanks. This is not a punishment. It is an experiment so you can gain a greater understanding of your patterns. After only a short period of time, you may see some patterns develop and thereby create a strategy to defeat a pattern of behavior that is keeping you from realizing your goal

PINPOINTING WHEN, WHERE, AND WHY YOU ARE EATING

The following exercise will help you to analyze your eating pattern.[13] When you go outside of the boundaries of *when* you should eat, or exceed the portion guidelines of *what* you should eat, your behavior patterns are standing in the way of your goal. To identify when you are most likely to use food, where you eat, and why you are eating, you will check yes or no for each item on the list below.

WHEN   **Yes**   **No**

When I ate at an unspecified time or overate, I felt:

	Yes	No
lonely	_____	_____
isolated	_____	_____
ignored	_____	_____
unhappy	_____	_____
stressed	_____	_____
insecure	_____	_____
awkward	_____	_____
uncomfortable	_____	_____
unimportant	_____	_____
Other:	_____	

WHERE   **Yes**   **No**

I ate: in the car   _____   _____

                                in front of the TV   _____   _____

                                at my desk   _____   _____

                                in employees' lounge   _____   _____

                                during commute   _____   _____

                                in a lounge or bar   _____   _____

                                at a social event   _____   _____

                                Other: _____

WHY   **Yes**   **No**

I ate because I needed: companionship   _____   _____

                                a break in the routine   _____   _____

                                comfort   _____   _____

                                relaxation   _____   _____

                                to be noticed   _____   _____

                                Other: _____

After you have pinpointed the times, locations, and reasons why you ate, you can begin to change your behavior pattern. Look back at the "When" category. Which ones are marked yes? In the chart below, under the "When" heading, write, "I ate when I was feeling [isolated, stressed, uncomfortable]." Follow the same procedure for the "Where" and "Why" categories. Now you should have three or more statements that ring true for you. (If they don't, review the items you have marked incorrectly.)

WHEN   **NEW OPTIONS**

_____   _____

_____   _____

_____   _____

_____   _____

WHERE   **NEW OPTIONS**

_____   _____

_____   _____

_____   _____

_____   _____

WHY   **NEW OPTIONS**

_____   _____

_____   _____

_____   _____

_____   _____

Now look at the "New Options" column. Don't fill this in immediately. Give yourself plenty of time to think of alternative activities or courses of action. Make sure that these new options genuinely appeal to you. Since they are the options that you will come to depend on as an alternative behavior during the next 6 months or one year, you need to stand behind them.

The following is an example of alternatives—new options for old habits.

WHEN	NEW OPTIONS
I ate when I was feeling isolated.	When I feel isolated, I will visit a friend, make a telephone call, write a letter, send an E-mail, offer to do something for someone else, or read a newspaper, magazine, or book.
I ate when I was feeling stressed.	When I feel stressed, I will close my eyes and breathe deeply 10 times, go for a walk, talk to someone about what is causing the immediate stress, or shift my attention to a constructive activity that I enjoy.

WHERE	NEW OPTIONS
I overate while driving.	While driving, I will breathe deeply and relax, concentrate on tightening and relaxing my muscles, or plan my next activity in detail.
I overate at a social event.	At social events, I will introduce myself to at least one unfamiliar person and carry on a short conversation. I will participate in discussions whenever the opportunity presents itself.

WHY	NEW OPTIONS
I ate when I needed a break in my routine.	If I need a break in my routine and I am engaged in a mental activity, I will change to a physical activity such as stretching, getting up for a short walk, chatting with someone, or getting some water.

GETTING THE SUPPORT YOU NEED

Because you will be using The Equation for an extended period of time, you may find it useful to seek more support than this book and your own resourcefulness can provide. The more allies you have, the better. You may choose to achieve your goal with a buddy or family member. You may seek counseling. You may decide to join a group of friends.

There are so many people who are going through this same exact thing right at this very moment. There is no reason why you should feel alone or isolated in achieving your goal. Because you will need support, it is our strong suggestion that you check out a group such as Overeaters Anonymous. Overeaters Anonymous has approximately 7,500 meeting groups in more than 50 countries.

Overeaters Anonymous

PO Box 44020

Rio Rancho, New Mexico 87124-4020

Telephone: (505) 891-2664

Fax: (505) 891-4320

E-mail: info@overeatersanonymous.org

REVERSING FAT GAIN AND HEALTH PROBLEMS

The primary concern is the amount of body fat you currently have and your strategy to reduce that amount of fat. But first you need to know how that fat came to be. When you were born, you came into this world with a certain amount of fat cells that were inherited. From the time you are born until the end of puberty, you can develop even more fat cells. You stop producing fat cells at the end of puberty, and from that point forward these fat cells can either grow or shrink. Fat cells can be shrunk down to fit several on the end of a pin, or they can grow to be the size of your head. Once you determine why this fat came to be and how you have enabled it to grow, you can go about the business of shrinking your fat cells.

OVERCOMING OBSTACLES

If you have been following each step in this book, you have made many positive and beneficial adjustments in your lifestyle to accommodate a shift in the way your particular body rids itself of fat.

This plan is an extreme form of getting results. To get the results you are looking for, you are going to be pushing the envelope. However, if you remain 50 or 100 pounds overweight much longer, there will be significant health problems down the line. Because your situation demands it, the time is *now* to make this change—but do it safely, quickly, and effectively. You will be doing this accelerated program for only 6 months or a year, so your goal is reachable. You only have to stay on course. Because this lifestyle shift is accelerated, you will have to become even more diligent about your nutritional guidelines and even more exacting in the number of calories you burn off.

All of us are different individuals, with differing needs and circumstances. All of us face challenges. There are obstacles that exist for you, and you should see them as factors that will challenge your will and desire. Obstacles and challenges can and will be overcome, but it is essential that they are at least acknowledged. There are three primary factors and three potential obstacles that all of us need to address: age, stress level, and time.

You need to realize that your age, your stress level, and your time have all been factors in putting on the weight you now want to lose. When we speak of lifestyle, and making adjustments, we are really talking about how to affect these three critical areas. If you are looking to lose 50 or more pounds, your age is certainly a factor in how that extra weight came to be. Take a look at your life over the last 5 or 10 years. Has your activity level slowed down at all? Whether you are 18 or 80, you can be more active than you are today. This does not mean that you need to be in training for a marathon, it just means that the more active you are the younger you will feel at any age.

Our level of stress and our time are directly linked to the number of responsibilities we have. The older we get, the more responsibilities we take on. It is quite possible that when you graduated from school you were much leaner than you are today. In those days, you had plenty of time for recreation. When you began a career or got married, that recreational time for activity was reduced. As you advanced in your work and/or had children, that recreational time spent on activity was diminished even further. The bottom line is that we all have responsibilities, and very often our last priority is ourselves. We would like to reiterate a simple profound truth: Your time is your own until you give it away. You can, in fact, reduce your level of stress by becoming more active. Even if it is a 15-minute walk, you will feel far less uptight when you are finished. Time is what you need to create. If you look carefully at your daily schedule, no matter how hectic or frenetic your pace, we guarantee you can find an hour in your day. This hour may typically be spent "relaxing." It may be an hour you watch television. It may be the hour you spend drinking coffee or reading the paper. It may be 10 minutes here and 30 minutes there, but somehow or other you can squeeze in an hour to fulfill your goal.

When you do find this hour, you shouldn't think of it as "selfish" time. Take a walk with someone close to you. Play with the kids or grandchildren. Spend that time doing helpful projects to improve your home or yard. Spend the time doing something you enjoy. Have fun. You deserve joy, and if you look at your activity as "having fun," chances are you will do more of it. If you can find some room in your life for a little bit more joy, you will have more to pass around to those you love. This time will be spent improving your life, and as a result, the quality of life of those you touch will be improved as well.

SUBSTITUTE, MODIFY, AND SHIFT

As always, the name of the game is staying on the plan. Staying on the plan does not mean that if you happen to fall that you cannot recover and get back on your feet. The Equation is relatively forgiving in that if you make a mistake there are many opportunities to make up for it. Still, at all times try to stay the course. There will be challenges and obstacles, but to a large degree there are three ways to effectively overcome those hurdles.

Whether you want to lose 50 or 100 pounds, you will have to adhere to the basic principle of The Equation. Meeting your goal is all about calories in and calories out. You will have to do everything in your power to make the commitment to create your own personal strategy and stick to it. If you are looking to adhere to your strategy and face obstacles that need to be overcome, your best options are to modify, substitute, or shift.

CUSTOMIZING "CALORIES IN"

The first step in personalizing The Equation comes with adjusting your food intake. To get the results you want, the first place to look should always be what is going into your mouth. Look over your body bills from last week to see exactly what you ate. Chances are that your new eating habits/lifestyle is a departure from what you had been doing in the past. How does this new lifestyle work for you? How is your energy? How is your level of hunger? Do you feel like you are depriving yourself? While you should give yourself a pat on the back for making these changes, you should also ask yourself some serious questions about how you may improve this level of refinement. In looking at your average day, is there a food or food group that you could substitute or modify? If you look at the foods at the top and at the bottom of the food guide pyramid, you can often identify problem areas. Are there alcoholic beverages that you could reduce or eliminate? Foods with high fat or sugar content that you could substitute or modify? How many times are you eating fast food? Could you make a shift in your lifestyle and eliminate fast food altogether? It is also possible that reducing your caloric intake has been difficult. The bottom line is that you have to find a way to make your "calories in" work for you.

Making it work means putting together a nutritional program that you can live with. What you have done up to this point is fantastic. Having many meals throughout the day and portioning them appropriately are the hard-and-fast rules, but only you can oversee what those meals and portions are.

If you are looking to retool your nutritional program, you will fall into one of four categories. We have given these four categories labels and created a game plan containing specific guidelines for each. *The Pushaway Artist* is a person who leaves 10 to 20 percent of his or her food on the plate. *The Specialty Artist* has dietary requirements such as being a vegetarian, or would like to implement a specific "diet." *The Weigher and Measurer* becomes extremely exacting about portions, weights, and sizes. *The Structured Personality* merely needs to be told exactly what to eat and when to eat it.

THE PUSHAWAY ARTIST

Becoming a Pushaway Artist is the easiest way to lose weight and the best way to insure a lifestyle that you enjoy. Most Pushaway Artists usually need to improve the types of foods they like, however, to insure getting all the nutrients and fiber the body needs. It is the easiest way to reduce your calories but does take some discipline.

Some people have the ability to eat only a certain amount of food and no more. Typically, these people always leave a significant portion of their meal on the plate. If you fall into this category, you have developed a fantastic habit, and this is not a time to become a person who "cleans his or her plate." Leaving food on your plate is a fantastic sign that you have the innate ability to eat only the food you need to satisfy you and not eat until you are "full." The distinction between satisfied and full is a great gift that you have developed, and it limits your course of action. The possibility that you are overeating is remote; therefore, the other two areas you should concentrate on are the caloric value of the foods you do eat and your level of activity.

Look at the food pyramid and notice the recommended daily servings for each food group. For example, it is suggested that you eat 6–11 portions from the grains group. Based on your weight on the scale, it is entirely possible that you do not need 11 starch servings per day. By accounting for your "calories in," you may balance your personal equation to get the results you are looking for.

In all likelihood, your area of concentration will be in looking at your caloric expenditure, the number of calories you are burning off each day. If you want to meet your goal, chances are that you need to increase your level of activity. If you have always wanted to take up a new sport or activity, now is the time. However, if you do not choose to do this, you should look at the activities you are already doing and do more of them or extend the length of time you are doing them.

If you fall in this category, make certain that you are within the guidelines for your caloric intake and also take a close look at the activity chart. By simply using the food pyramid/food list, and by accumulating credits by additional activity, you should meet your goal without any difficulty.

THE SPECIALTY ARTIST

Hollywood is filled with Specialty Artists. Specialty Artists use The Equation to create a way of eating they believe is best, most effective, and healthy for their lifestyles. Specialty Artists create food patterns they believe are best to help them lose fat and improve health, energy, and well-being. People who follow a specific plan like a high-protein or low-carbohydrate food plan are Specialty Artists.

The Specialty Artist requires a specific set of guidelines for his or her nutritional program. The Specialty Artist may be a vegetarian who will not or cannot eat meat. He or she may prefer a high-protein diet, a high-carbohydrate diet, a low-carbohydrate diet, a no-sugar/no-carbohydrate diet, or some structured regimen that already exists.

Be assured that if you fall into this category, you may use any "diet" that you choose. The Equation will provide the necessary layer to help you achieve your goal on time. Again, no matter what the diet, anyone who has ever had success reduced his or her caloric intake, or increased his or her level of activity, or a combination of both. By using The Equation, you will become exacting about the calories you take in and the calories you burn off through activity. If you fall into this category, you should use the food pyramid and the corresponding food lists to create your own personal equation. In conjunction with your own special eating regimen, you will get the results you desire and meet your goals.

THE WEIGHER AND MEASURER

In Hollywood, the Weigher and Measurer usually is the star's chef; however, many celebrities have become quite good at knowing how to estimate the calories of food through association by having weighed the food or actually used a measuring cup to exactly determine an amount of food or liquid. A Weigher and Measurer is also good at checking labels and is able to add up calories. He or she is able to closely estimate the number of calories taken in throughout the day.

Some of us are very exacting. The Weigher and Measurer is precise about the number of calories he or she takes in and also the number of calories he or she is burning off. Typically this type of person has the greatest results because he or she is so specific and so focused on getting the desired results.

If you fall into this category, simply follow the food lists and activity chart, and you are guaranteed the greatest possible chance of meeting your goal.

THE STRUCTURED PERSONALITY

This type of person is really one who likes to follow a guide. Most of us have followed a food guideline. Food guidelines can be specific with recipes that cater to certain interests or they can be used as a general guideline to follow. Many people like to be accountable to a guideline. This structure can be very successful in helping people establish a new healthy habit or they can be used with people who don't mind following a game plan. Athletes are often used to following a game plan, knowing that it is a part of reaching the goal. Over time this is the hardest to maintain, because it is best used for short-term results.

Some people just want the answers. They can't be bothered by the details, they just need to be told what to do, and they will follow the instructions to the letter. They do not have the time, energy, or interest to structure their own personalized program but are able to take a structured eating regimen and use it with no problem at all.

If you fall into this category, we have included an example of a nutritionally correct 1,800-calorie program for you to follow. If you actually need exactly 1,800 calories per day, you are in luck. If you require more calories, choose foods from the food list (attached to the food pyramid) and add the number of calories you need to each meal. If you need fewer calories per meal, use the foods listed as a guideline by reducing the quantity of them.

This example of a nutritional plan has been formulated to meet the daily recommended intake levels for all vitamins and minerals. Targeted percent intakes of some vitamins and minerals exceed the 100 percent in an attempt to optimize the intake of these microingredients. Additionally, percent of caloric intake has been targeted for an approximate intake of 55–60 percent carbohydrate, 15–20 percent protein, and 30 percent or less fat.

As with any nutritional program or change in health behavior, you should consult with your physician, prior to participation, to evaluate this nutritional guideline and confirm that it is appropriate for you based on your individual needs and requirements.[14]

91% 3 1800 =
       1648

DAY 1

BREAKFAST	¾ cup Cheerios, ½ cup skim milk, 1 banana
A.M. SNACK	1 cup orange juice, ½ grapefruit
LUNCH	2 ounces tuna salad on whole wheat bread, 2 slices tomato, lettuce, 1 slice Cheddar cheese
P.M. SNACK	1 cup fruit yogurt, 2 graham crackers
DINNER	3 ounces chicken breast, 1 cup white rice, ½ cup black beans, salad with tomato and carrot, vinegar/oil dressing

---

DAY 2

BREAKFAST	1 packet instant oatmeal, 1 cup skim milk, ½ grapefruit
A.M. SNACK	½ small bagel, ½ tablespoon cream cheese, ½ cup tomato juice
LUNCH	3 ounces turkey sandwich with 2 slices tomato on wheat bread, 1 slice cheese, lettuce
P.M. SNACK	¾ cup low-fat fruit yogurt, 2 plain granola bars
DINNER	4 ounces steamed salmon, ½ cup brown rice, 1 cup broccoli, 1 cup tea

---

DAY 3

BREAKFAST	¾ cup Multigrain Cheerios, 1 cup skim milk, ½ grapefruit
A.M. SNACK	1 banana, ½ cup cottage cheese
LUNCH	4 ounces hamburger, 2 slices wheat bread, 2 slices tomato, lettuce, 1 cup skim milk
P.M. SNACK	2 nonfat fig bar cookies, ¼ cantaloupe
DINNER	3 ounces baked cod, 5 tablespoons green beans, baked potato, 1 tablespoon margarine, 2 slices wheat bread, 1 cup skim milk

DAY 4

BREAKFAST	¾ cup Total cereal, 1 cup skim milk, ½ cup orange juice
A.M. SNACK	1 small orange, 1 granola bar
LUNCH	4-ounce grilled chicken breast sandwich on white bread, 1 cup green salad, 1 ounce oil/vinegar dressing
P.M. SNACK	1 cup fruit cocktail, 1 tablespoon granola cereal
DINNER	4-ounce tuna filet, ½ cup steamed carrots, salad with tomatoes, low-cal French dressing, 1 cup white rice, 1 slice multigrain bread, 2 graham crackers, 1 peach, 1 cup skim milk

DAY 5

BREAKFAST	1 small bran muffin, 1 cup skim milk, ½ cup strawberries
A.M. SNACK	¾ cup fruit yogurt
LUNCH	3-ounce chicken taco with tomato slices, ½ cup black beans, 1 cup skim milk
P.M. SNACK	1 banana, 1 orange, 1 plain bagel
DINNER	3-ounce baked salmon, 5 tablespoons peas, ½ cup brown rice, leaf lettuce with cucumber slices and oil/vinegar dressing, 2 slices French bread, 1 cup tea

DAY 6

BREAKFAST	¾ cup Multigrain Cheerios, 1 cup skim milk, ½ cup orange juice
A.M. SNACK	2 graham crackers, 1 apple, 2 ounces Cheddar cheese
LUNCH	1 cup pasta salad with ½ cup broccoli, sliced half tomato, light oil; 1 cup fruit juice
P.M. SNACK	¾ cup fruit yogurt, flour tortilla
DINNER	4 ounces roast beef, baked potato, 1 tablespoon butter, 5 tablespoons green beans, salad with tomato slices and low-cal Italian dressing, 4 pieces melba toast, 1 cup tea

DAY 7

BREAKFAST	1 small bran muffin, 1 piece cracked wheat toast, ½ grapefruit, ½ cup fruit juice, 1 cup skim milk
A.M. SNACK	8 Triscuit crackers, ½ carrot, 1 slice cheese, 1 cup skim milk
LUNCH	3 ounces turkey on 2 slices wheat bread, lettuce and 2 slices tomato, 1 banana
P.M. SNACK	¾ cup fruit yogurt
DINNER	4-ounce center-cut pork filet, ½ cup white rice, ½ cup green beans, salad with tomato and 1 teaspoon low-cal French dressing

WEEK 2

DAY 1

BREAKFAST	1 cup Total cereal, 1 cup skim milk
A.M. SNACK	½ cup strawberries, 2 graham crackers
LUNCH	1 cup instant vegetable soup, 10 Wheat Thin crackers, 3 ounces Colby cheese, 1 apple
P.M. SNACK	1 banana, 1 cup low-fat yogurt
DINNER	1 cup turkey chili, salad with 5 cucumber slices, 1 tablespoon Parmesan cheese, light salad dressing, 2 slices Italian bread, 1 tablespoon butter, 1 cup tea

DAY 2

BREAKFAST	3 silver dollar (5-inch) pancakes, 3 tablespoons light syrup, ½ cup cranberry juice, 1 cup skim milk
A.M. SNACK	sliced celery and carrots, 10 Wheat Thins
LUNCH	1 turkey and ham lunch meat sandwich on rye bread, 1 slice cheese, 2 tomatoes, 1 lettuce leaf, 1 diet soda
P.M. SNACK	2 fat-free fig bar cookies
DINNER	3 ounces baked salmon, ½ cup broccoli, 4 new potatoes, salad with light oil dressing, 1 slice French bread, 1 cup tea

DAY 3

BREAKFAST	1 bran muffin, 1 grapefruit, 1 cup skim milk, ½ cup orange juice
A.M. SNACK	1 plain bagel, 5 tablespoons cream cheese
LUNCH	1 cup fruit salad with 1 cup vanilla yogurt, 2 lettuce leaves, 1 wheat roll, 1 slice wheat bread, 1 teaspoon butter, 1 diet soda
P.M. SNACK	1 banana, 2 ounces cheese, 10 Wheat Thins
DINNER	1 cup pasta with 1 cup meat/tomato sauce, 5 tablespoons green beans, salad with 2 tablespoons green peppers, 1 tablespoon Parmesan cheese, 1 tablespoon low-cal Italian dressing, 1 cup tea

DAY 4

BREAKFAST	1 cup Total cereal, 1 banana, 1 cup skim milk
A.M. SNACK	8 Wheat Thins, 1 slice cheese, ½ cup fruit juice
LUNCH	½ cup turkey chili, 4 pieces melba toast, 1 apple, 1 flavored seltzer
P.M. SNACK	5 carrot sticks and celery sticks, 2 low-fat fig bars, 1 cup low-fat fruit yogurt
DINNER	3 ounces baked chicken breast, 5 tablespoons broccoli, ½ cup white rice, salad with ½ sliced tomato, 2 tablespoons sweet green peppers, oil/vinegar dressing

DAY 5

BREAKFAST	1 cup Multigrain Cheerios, 1 cup skim milk, ½ cup cranberry juice
A.M. SNACK	4 graham crackers, 1 banana
LUNCH	turkey breast lunch meat on wheat bread, 1 slice provolone cheese, 1 lettuce leaf, 2 slices tomato, 1 diet soda
P.M. SNACK	8 Triscuit crackers, ½ cup cottage cheese, 1 apple
DINNER	4 ounces cod, ½ cup brown rice, 5 tablespoons green beans, salad with 4 tomato slices and 1 tablespoon low-cal Italian dressing, 1 cup low-fat fruit yogurt

DAY 6

BREAKFAST	2 waffles with fruit jam, 1 cup skim milk, ½ cup fruit juice
A.M. SNACK	1 apple, 8 whole wheat crackers
LUNCH	2 ounces tuna salad on whole wheat bread with 2 lettuce leaves, 1 slice Monterey Jack cheese, 1 cup skim milk
P.M. SNACK	1 banana, 1 granola bar
DINNER	3 ounces turkey, baked potato, 5 tablespoons broccoli, salad with 8 tomato slices, 1 slice French bread

DAY 7

BREAKFAST	1 English muffin with jam, 1 cup skim milk, ½ cup orange juice
A.M. SNACK	1 granola bar, 1 banana
LUNCH	1 turkey breast lunch meat sandwich on whole wheat bread, light mustard, 2 lettuce leaves, 2 slices tomato, 1 slice cheese, 1 twisted pretzel, 2 cups skim milk
P.M. SNACK	2 graham crackers, 1 apple
DINNER	½ cup pasta with 2 tablespoons sauce, 2 ounces chicken breast, salad with tomatoes and light oil dressing

WEEK 3

DAY 1

BREAKFAST	½ cup granola cereal, 1 cup skim milk, 1 banana
A.M. SNACK	¾ cup fruit yogurt
LUNCH	4 ounces hamburger, ½ cup pasta salad, 1 slice tomato, 1 lettuce leaf, 1 diet soda
P.M. SNACK	1 apple, 5 Triscuits
DINNER	3-ounce tuna filet, ½ cup brown rice, 5 tablespoons green beans, 2 tablespoons carrots, salad with cucumber with ranch-type dressing, 1 cup tea

---

DAY 2

Breakfast	2 slices French toast with 1 tablespoon light syrup, 1 cup skim milk, ½ cup orange juice
a.m. Snack	4 ounces fruit cup, 2 graham crackers
Lunch	1 cup fruit salad, 6 lettuce leaves, 10 Triscuits, ½ cup cottage cheese
p.m. Snack	1 cup applesauce, 2 granola bars
Dinner	3 ounces baked salmon, small baked potato, ½ tablespoon butter, 4 tablespoons peas, salad with 1 chopped small tomato and 1 teaspoon carrots, 1 tablespoon low-cal French dressing

---

DAY 3

Breakfast	1 cup Total, 1 banana, 1 cup skim milk, ½ cup orange juice
a.m. Snack	1 cup fruit yogurt, 2 graham crackers
Lunch	2 slices cheese pizza
p.m. Snack	5 carrot sticks, 2 graham crackers
Dinner	1 large baked potato with ½ tablespoon butter, ½ cup broccoli, 1 tablespoon shredded cheese, salad with tomatoes and 2 tablespoons low-cal mayo-type dressing

---

DAY 4

Breakfast	1 English muffin, light jam, 1 cup skim milk, 1 cup apple juice
a.m. Snack	4 ounces fruit cup, 2 graham crackers
Lunch	1 chicken taco with lettuce, tomatoes, and 2 tablespoons shredded cheese; 1 cup skim milk
p.m. Snack	1 apple, 8 sesame crackers, 1 ounce Cheddar cheese
Dinner	1 cup pasta with 2 tablespoons tomato/meat sauce, 1 tablespoon Parmesan cheese, salad with tomato and carrot and 1 tablespoon light oil dressing, 1 cup tea

---

DAY 5

BREAKFAST	1 English muffin, light jam, 1 cup skim milk, ½ cup orange juice
A.M. SNACK	2 flour tortillas, 1 slice cheese
LUNCH	1 cup ramen noodle soup, 1 apple
P.M. SNACK	1 granola bar, 1 cup low-fat fruit yogurt
DINNER	½ cup minestrone soup, salad with cucumbers and 1 tablespoon vinegar-oil or low-cal mayo-type dressing, 2 slices mixed grain bread, ½ teaspoon butter

---

DAY 6

BREAKFAST	¾ cup Cheerios, 1 cup skim milk, 1 banana
A.M. SNACK	1 cup strawberries, 1 cup vanilla yogurt, 2 graham crackers
LUNCH	1 small baked potato, 5 tablespoons broccoli, 2 slices rye bread, 1 cup skim milk
P.M. SNACK	1 plain bagel
DINNER	3 ounces broiled veal, 4 small new potatoes, 5 tablespoons corn, ¼ cup brown rice, salad with light oil dressing

---

DAY 7

BREAKFAST	1 small bagel, ½ cup strawberries, 1 cup skim milk
A.M. SNACK	2 flour tortillas, 5 carrot sticks, ½ cup fruit yogurt
LUNCH	3-ounce ham sandwich on rye bread, 1 slice cheese, 2 slices tomato, 2 lettuce leaves, mustard, 1 apple, 1 cup skim milk
P.M. SNACK	1 cup applesauce, 2 graham crackers
DINNER	4 ounces baked salmon, 5 tablespoons green beans, 4 new potatoes, salad with oil/vinegar dressing

WEEK 4

DAY 1

BREAKFAST	1 bagel, light jam, ½ grapefruit, 1 cup skim milk, 1 cup apple juice
A.M. SNACK	2 graham crackers, 1 cup fruit salad
LUNCH	10 Triscuits, turkey sandwich with light mayo or mustard on rye bread, 1 slice cheese, 1 cup skim milk
P.M. SNACK	¾ cup fruit yogurt, 2 graham crackers
DINNER	1 cup pasta with tomato/meat sauce, 3 tablespoons green beans, salad with cucumbers, 2 slices French bread, ¼ tablespoon butter, 2 ounces fruit salad, 1 cup skim milk

---

DAY 2

BREAKFAST	2 slices wheat toast, 2 teaspoons butter, light jam, 1 banana, 1 cup skim milk, 10 ounces apple juice
A.M. SNACK	¼ cantaloupe
LUNCH	leafy green salad with tomato slices, cucumbers, and 1 tablespoon shredded carrot; 2 slices cheese, 8 Wheat Thins, 1 cup skim milk
P.M. SNACK	1 apple, 1 banana
DINNER	3 ounces poached chicken breast, 1 baked potato, 1 tablespoon butter, 4 tablespoons peas, 4 ounces fruit cup, 1 cup tea

---

DAY 3

BREAKFAST	1 cup Total, 1 banana, 1 cup skim milk, 10 ounces apple juice
A.M. SNACK	2 flour tortillas, 1 cup water
LUNCH	1 ham/turkey sandwich on wheat bread, 1 slice cheese, 2 tomato slices, 2 lettuce leaves
P.M. SNACK	2 graham crackers, 4 ounces fruit cup
DINNER	3 ounces veal, 5 new potatoes, 4 tablespoons green beans, salad with tomato and 1 tablespoon oil dressing

---

DAY 4

BREAKFAST	1 bran muffin, 1 cup skim milk, 10 ounces apple juice
A.M. SNACK	4 ounces fruit cup with 1 cup vanilla yogurt, 10 Triscuits
LUNCH	1 chicken breast sandwich, 1 slice tomato, 1 lettuce leaf, 1 slice cheese
P.M. SNACK	1 cup microwave or air-popped popcorn, 1 diet soda
DINNER	1 cup pasta with 2 tablespoons sauce, 4-ounce chicken breast, 5 tablespoons green beans, 2 teaspoons Parmesan cheese

---

DAY 5

BREAKFAST	1 cup Cheerios, 1 cup skim milk, 10 ounces cranberry juice
A.M. SNACK	1 grapefruit
LUNCH	2 slices cheese pizza, 4 ounces fruit salad
P.M. SNACK	2 ounces pretzel thins, ½ cup cottage cheese
DINNER	1 cup white rice, 3 tablespoons green beans, 4 pieces broccoli, salad with tomatoes and 1 tablespoon light dressing, 2 slices French bread, ⅓ tablespoon butter

---

DAY 6

BREAKFAST	1 English muffin, light jam, 1 cup skim milk, 10 ounces juice
A.M. Snack	½ grapefruit, 8 Wheat Thins
LUNCH	fruit salad with lettuce, ½ cup cottage cheese, 1 slice cheese, 2 ounces tuna salad with light mayo
P.M. SNACK	1 cup fruit yogurt, 8 Triscuits
DINNER	3 ounces baked cod, 1 cup brown rice, 4 tablespoons carrots, 1 tablespoon oil/vinegar dressing

DAY 7

Breakfast	1 cup raisin bran cereal, 1 cup milk, ½ cup strawberries, 10 ounces juice
a.m. Snack	8 graham crackers, 1 tablespoon peanut butter
Lunch	3-ounce turkey sandwich on whole wheat bread with lettuce and 2 slices cheese, 1 cup milk
p.m. Snack	4 ounces fruit cup and 1 cup vanilla yogurt
Dinner	1 cup pasta with tomato sauce, 1 tablespoon Parmesan cheese, salad with tomatoes and light French dressing

YOUR STRATEGY TO LOSE 50 POUNDS OR MORE

If you have chosen this plan because you have 50 pounds of fat to lose, there are a number of issues that warrant serious discussion. First and foremost, you have health concerns that are going to become more serious if you do not address them soon. Before you begin this program, you should consult with a doctor to determine what kind of exercise might be most appropriate for you. The health concerns that you are facing right now, or will face in the future, should be a major motivating factor to improve your current condition. Help is on the way.

The most critical issue to address is the way you are using food. More specifically, you are using food as an emotional crutch much like alcoholics use alcohol and drug addicts use drugs. When confronted with the possibility of addiction, those who are addicted have a tendency to deny their problem. For your sake, please do not ignore the possiblity, but rather entertain it and see if you answer yes to the following questions. Do you ever eat to make yourself feel better? Are stressful occasions followed by a large meal or binge eating? Like people who have drinking buddies, do you have one or more friends that you can really eat with? Most people who have 50 or more pounds to lose are eating emotionally, and this behavior needs to be modified in order for you to see any significant changes.

A number of factors are involved in your particular situation, but your weight-loss issues are mostly behavioral concerns. There is a certain amount of imbalance present in your life, and these imbalances have to be addressed as well. In some cases there is an interruption of the basic cycles of life. You may be sleeping more hours than you are awake, or you may be sleeping in the daytime and are awake at night. Essentially, your daily schedule is in a place of imbalance. More frequently, responsibilities and the inability to cope with your stresses have interrupted your daily balance.

We can state with some certainty that you are not exercising. (If you exercise at least 4 times per week, my guess is that there may be some medical explanation for the condition you would like to reverse.) Your work begins here. We would like you to exercise for at least 30 consecutive minutes per day. During this exercise period, be focused upon your heart rate and if possible use a heart-rate monitor to make certain you stay within the boundaries of performance. Estimate your training range by subtracting your age from 220. This number reflects your maximum heart rate. You should never, ever reach this number while exercising. Now divide your maximum heart rate by 2, or 50 percent. For the first 2 weeks try to walk 30 consecutive minutes each and every day, and make certain that your heart is beating at 50 percent of your maximum heart rate. The second 2 weeks, reach 60 percent of your maximum heart rate for 30 minutes, then 70 percent for the remainder of your program. Increase the long duration of those walks as it becomes more comfortable. You will be surprised how little effort increases your heart rate to 50 percent. It is quite possible that just walking will suit your needs. As you increase your heart rate, you may find that more exaggerated arm movements will get you up to 60 percent. As you reach 70 percent, you may find it helpful to have access to exercise equipment such as a stationary bike, elliptical trainer, or a stair climber found at the gym.

When Tom Hanks was shooting *Philadelphia*, he played a lawyer with AIDS whose condition grew worse throughout the film. The film was shot in progression, meaning that they shot the first scene of the movie and filmed sequentially until they finished the script. In each scene, Tom Hanks would have to appear thinner as a result of the illness. Each week, Tom had to be 2½ pounds lighter. In all, Tom Hanks lost about 40 pounds in four months.

It may not be possible or comfortable for you to use aerobic exercises at this very moment, but it is essential to do something. When we discussed The Equation, we talked about many levels of "balance." The level that is the biggest concern for you is the balance between lean muscle mass and body fat. We have not suggested strength training at any other stage of this book, but weight-bearing exercises will have significant benefits for you. If you can increase your percentage of lean muscle mass, you will consequently reduce your percentage of body fat. As a result of this increase in lean muscle mass you will burn more calories throughout the day. There is nothing more beneficial for you than beginning a strength-training program.

Light aerobic activity is introduced into your equation almost immediately, and you should increase that activity every week until you are halfway to your goal. In addition to daily exercise, we suggest that you partake in strength-training exercises when you are halfway to your goal. Begin by using strength-training exercises 3 days per week. After a month or 6 weeks, try to increase to 4 days per week. At this point, you would be doing at least 40 minutes of aerobic activity per day and participating in strength training at least 4 times per week. You will only need to maintain this program or increase the duration of aerobic sessions to exceed your goal.

With your exercise program firmly in place, it is time to address your issues of emotional eating. There are many foods that you consider "comfort foods." These foods are either sweetened with sugar, high in fat content, or both. These are the foods you want to try to reduce or eliminate from your diet. You might find that you handle stress with a half-gallon of ice cream, or a cake, or doughnuts, or breads, or potatoes, or food your grandmother cooked. These foods are not giving you true comfort. When you look at yourself in the mirror, these foods are actually making you miserable. When you eat sugar, you will crave more sugar throughout the day. If you have a doughnut for breakfast, you are setting yourself up to crave more and more sugar throughout the day. Remember, carbohydrates are just the same as sugar, so there are similar cravings with bread, potatoes, and pasta. You need to find ways to replace these foods. Instead of ice cream, you may find that a chocolate tofu mousse satisfies your craving. You may find that chewing sugar-free gum after meals abates these cravings. You may discover that eating a greater percentage of protein in each meal makes you feel full and less likely to crave sugars and carbohydrates.

If you have followed the suggestions in Chapters 2 through 5 to the letter, you have accomplished much in modifying the behaviors that have led you to put on weight. Using all of those strategies, you are going to make only small adjustments to your eating program. The first meal of the day is especially important for you. The number of meals is also crucial. Rather than eating out of hunger, you crave food for other reasons. We suspect that you would rather have your entire allotment of daily calories in one sitting than spaced throughout the day. You probably were not eating frequently enough before you began reading this book, and the frequency of your meals is vital to your success. After breakfast, your meals should have a high content of vegetables. Again, your objective is to avoid foods with a high sugar content. The higher the fiber content of your vegetables, the better. When and if you do eat carbohydrates, it is important to have little or no additional fat in your meal. When there is too much glucose in your bloodstream, insulin is secreted. Insulin has one job: to take excess glucose and place it within your fat cells. When fat is present in your diet, the fat molecules are often attached to glucose molecules and both are placed within the fat cell.

YOUR GAME PLAN

1. Make 365 copies of the daily worksheet (page 114). Place these in a binder, day-planner, or journal. Take this wherever you go.
2. Make at least 20 copies of the When, Where, and Why sheet (page 148) and place this in your journal. When you go outside the guidelines of The Equation, fill out the sheet.
3. Make 26 copies of the Your Personal Equation worksheet (page 127). Every 2 weeks you will need to refigure your personal equation.
4. Week 1 marks the start of your activity program. If possible, each

day should include 30 minutes of continuous aerobic activity at 50 percent of your maximum heart rate. Week 2 you will increase to 60 percent. You can increase the duration of your walks up to 60 minutes if it is comfortable for you.

5. Weigh yourself only once a week to check your progress. Have your body fat measured every 2 weeks or at least every month to get a total picture of your success.

6. If your obstacles seem too great, get more support.

7. When you are halfway to your goal, start our strength-training program. With strength training you are creating lean muscle mass and automatically decreasing your body-fat percentage.

8. Place a small notebook on your refrigerator. Any time you find yourself opening the fridge and just peering in, stop and think about why you are doing this. Contemplate what you are feeling at this exact moment and write those feelings on the notepad.

EQUATION CREDIT CALENDAR

DAY 1	DAY 2	DAY 3	DAY 4	DAY 5	DAY 6	DAY 7
1 Calories in–3 Calories out–2 Total–5	2 Calories in–3 Calories out–2 Total–5	3 Calories in–3 Calories out–2 Total–5	4 Calories in–3 Calories out–3 Total–6	5 Calories in–3 Calories out–3 Total–6	6 Calories in–3 Calories out–3 Total–6	7 Calories in–3 Calories out–3 Total–6 Total Week–39
8 Calories in–3 Calories out–2 Total–5	9 Calories in–3 Calories out–2 Total–5	10 Calories in–3 Calories out–2 Total–5	11 Calories in–3 Calories out–3 Total–6	12 Calories in–3 Calories out–3 Total–6	13 Calories in–3 Calories out–3 Total–6	14 Calories in–3 Calories out–3 Total–6 Total Week–39
15 Calories in–3 Calories out–2 Total–5	16 Calories in–3 Calories out–2 Total–5	17 Calories in–3 Calories out–2 Total–5	18 Calories in–3 Calories out–3 Total–6	19 Calories in–3 Calories out–3 Total–6	20 Calories in–3 Calories out–3 Total–6	21 Calories in–3 Calories out–3 Total–6 Total Week–39
22 Calories in–3 Calories out–2 Total–5	23 Calories in–3 Calories out–2 Total–5	24 Calories in–3 Calories out–3 Total–6	25 Calories in–3 Calories out–3 Total–6	26 Calories in–3 Calories out–3 Total–6	27 Calories in–3 Calories out–3 Total–6	28 Calories in–3 Calories out–3 Total–6 Total Week–40
29 Calories in–3 Calories out–3 Total–6	30 Calories in–3 Calories out–3 Total–6	31 Calories in–3 Calories out–3 Total–6 Total Week–18				Total Month–175 Total Fat Loss– 5 pounds

EQUATION CREDIT CALENDAR

DAY 1	DAY 2	DAY 3	DAY 4	DAY 5	DAY 6	DAY 7
1 Calories in–4 Calories out–5 Total–9	2 Calories in–4 Calories out–5 Total–9	3 Calories in–4 Calories out–5 Total–9	4 Calories in–4 Calories out–5 Total–9	5 Calories in–4 Calories out–5 Total–9	6 Calories in–4 Calories out–5 Total–9	7 Calories in–4 Calories out–5 Total–9 Total Week–63
8 Calories in–4 Calories out–5 Total–9	9 Calories in–4 Calories out–5 Total–9	10 Calories in–4 Calories out–5 Total–9	11 Calories in–4 Calories out–5 Total–9	12 Calories in–4 Calories out–5 Total–9	13 Calories in–4 Calories out–5 Total–9	14 Calories in–4 Calories out–5 Total–9 Total Week–63
15 Calories in–4 Calories out–5 Total–9	16 Calories in–4 Calories out–5 Total–9	17 Calories in–4 Calories out–5 Total–9	18 Calories in–4 Calories out–5 Total–9	19 Calories in–4 Calories out–5 Total–9	20 Calories in–4 Calories out–5 Total–9	21 Calories in–4 Calories out–5 Total–9 Total Week–63
22 Calories in–4 Calories out–5 Total–9	23 Calories in–4 Calories out–5 Total–9	24 Calories in–4 Calories out–5 Total–9	25 Calories in–4 Calories out–5 Total–9	26 Calories in–4 Calories out–5 Total–9	27 Calories in–4 Calories out–5 Total–9	28 Calories in–4 Calories out–5 Total–9 Total Week–63
29 Calories in–4 Calories out–5 Total–9	30 Calories in–4 Calories out–5 Total–9	31 Calories in–4 Calories out–5 Total–9 Total Week–27			Total Month–279	Total Fat Loss– 8 pounds

EQUATION CREDIT CALENDAR

DAY 1	DAY 2	DAY 3	DAY 4	DAY 5	DAY 6	DAY 7
1 Calories in– Calories out– Total–	2 Calories in– Calories out– Total–	3 Calories in– Calories out– Total–	4 Calories in– Calories out– Total–	5 Calories in– Calories out– Total–	6 Calories in– Calories out– Total–	7 Calories in– Calories out– Total– Total Week–
8 Calories in– Calories out– Total–	9 Calories in– Calories out– Total–	10 Calories in– Calories out– Total–	11 Calories in– Calories out– Total–	12 Calories in– Calories out– Total–	13 Calories in– Calories out– Total–	14 Calories in– Calories out– Total– Total Week–
15 Calories in– Calories out– Total–	16 Calories in– Calories out– Total–	17 Calories in– Calories out– Total–	18 Calories in– Calories out– Total–	19 Calories in– Calories out– Total–	20 Calories in– Calories out– Total–	21 Calories in– Calories out– Total– Total Week–
22 Calories in– Calories out– Total–	23 Calories in– Calories out– Total–	24 Calories in– Calories out– Total–	25 Calories in– Calories out– Total–	26 Calories in– Calories out– Total–	27 Calories in– Calories out– Total–	28 Calories in– Calories out– Total– Total Week–
29 Calories in– Calories out– Total–	30 Calories in– Calories out– Total–	31 Calories in– Calories out– Total– Total Week–				Total Month– Total Fat Loss– ___ pounds

PART FIVE

EQUATION

for

MAINTENANCE

CHAPTER TWELVE

Equation for Lasting Results

This chapter is about maintaining your results. You have worked very hard to achieve the tremendous results you are now enjoying. You have been diligent and vigilant about what you have put into your body, and you have made great strides to become more and more active. Along with small lifestyle changes, these have been the key areas that have gotten you to this point. You have heard the old saying a hundred times, "If it ain't broke, don't fix it," and it is critical that you attempt to keep these new habits intact. As you have now discovered, your new lifestyle has paid incredible dividends, and if you can maintain these habits for 18 months, they will pay off throughout your life. Again it is important to stress that it is far more beneficial to make lasting results than to opt for the quick fix.

The greatest strategy to maintain your results is to continue doing exactly what you have been doing. By combining a proper intake of water with an eating schedule that includes five small meals per day (beginning within an hour after you wake up and every 2½ to 3 hours) and doing more of the activities you are already doing, you can and will maintain the results you have achieved. These habits will become a part of your new persona, and you will regard them as part of your regular regimen. If you find yourself reverting back to old habits, it is important that you acknowledge the pattern as quickly as possible and correct your course.

In a very profound sense, the end of this book is really the beginning, and the beginning is the end. In other words, water intake, the timing of your meals, the size of your portions, the amount of calories you take and the amount of calories you expend will always be the variables you are working with. This will never change. When these elements are all in place you can and will maintain the results you achieved and can even continue to achieve new results. Maintenance is about being and remaining vigilant with your new lifestyle.

YOUR COMFORT ZONE

Each of us has what we call a "comfort zone." There is a weight and body-fat percentage at which our body prefers to be. In meeting your goal, it is quite possible that you have gone below that comfort zone, and your body will unconsciously try to take you back to a level that is more comfortable. Often our comfort zone and our body's comfort zone are two distinctly different ideals.

Your body's comfort zone is an important factor in maintaining your results. We all have a natural tendency to revert back on behavior that we are comfortable with. By imposing your goals onto the level of body fat your body is most comfortable at, you have thrown your body into a state of confusion. Take a look at the composition of your body. Where there once was a great deal more body fat, there is now less of it. Nerves, the electrical impulses, and your metabolism all were used to your previous amount of fat, and without it, your body is not functioning as it is used to. When it is confused, it wants to go back to what it knows. You may find yourself unconsciously eating sweets and chocolates, you may find yourself eating large meals. Just be aware that it is your body wanting to get back to a level that it is comfortable with. In a situation such as this, you must consciously exert your will to rule your body's unconscious tendencies.

It takes some time for your body to adjust to this change, the "new you." It is usually a matter of months—not years—before this new normal is accepted by your body. During those months it is vital to combat your body's natural tendencies toward putting fat and weight back on. To do this it is essential that you increase your level of activity. Perhaps you are so excited about the changes that you want to take your physical transformation even farther. Perhaps you now have new goals, like trying to see your abdominal muscles, or getting into your wedding dress, or fitting into your "really skinny clothes." You may have increased your activity level to such a degree that you want to take up a sport, or train for a marathon, or try to get into a body-building contest. What would be the harm in that? You would only get yourself in better shape, and with maintenance, you could take your transformation still farther. There are so many things that you can do, and so many directions in which to take your transformation. If you achieved your goals using Chapters 2 through 4, you may want to explore the addition of regular exercise. If you determined that Chapter 7 or 8 suited your needs, and found that you achieved your goal, you may want to strongly consider embarking on a strength-training program. By taking full advantage of the "new you" and building on the momentum you have already created, you can and will offset any natural propensity to regain the fat, weight, and inches you have lost. Strength training and aerobic activity are important in reinforcing the changes you have made, allowing these changes to take root, and even propelling you toward new goals.

EACH DECADE IS A NEW CHALLENGE

Not only have you developed behavioral and lifestyle changes that have enabled you to become leaner, but these new lifestyle changes have also decreased your chances for disease and, potentially, will give you a greater life expectancy.

For each decade of life, we have new health issues that are increasingly important to us as time passes. What we eat and how we move are critical components of this process. By the time we reach puberty we have developed all the fat cells we will have for the rest of our lives. In our teens and twenties, we are establishing lifestyle choices and behaviors that will help us to stay lean or add body fat. In our mid to late twenties, we usually are getting married, settling into our adult lives, and thinking about if not having children. Most of this age group is no longer in school and is spending far less time engaged in physical activity.

In our thirties, we are taking on heavier responsibilities with work and family, and that generally means we are spending less time on ourselves and not maintaining our bodies with either proper nutrition or regular exercise. For this stage, and all others that follow, it is essential that we increase the amount of regular exercise. There is almost a panic about the level of exercise in children, but we are much more concerned about the number of people over 35 who are engaged in little or no exercise. The older we get, the more important exercise becomes. The late thirties and all of our forties are really our most productive time in the workplace. We are reaching the top of our professions, we are thinking about and working toward a day when we will retire, we are planning for the long term, and we have reached some understanding of our own mortality. If we haven't begun to make room in our lives to take good care of our bodies by this stage of our lives, the clock begins ticking toward a wake-up call.

In our fifties, we reach a critical mass. If we have failed to take time for proper nutrition and regular exercise, generally we will be scared into doing so as a direct result of "the wake-up call" or medical problems we encounter. What we are doing by the time we reach 55 is critical in the aging process. If we are exercising regularly and are on a great nutritional program, we will have the appearance of aging only 5 years in the next 15. If we do not, we will look 15 years older within the next 5. In our sixties, our vitality depends more on our activity level than any other factor. If we can increase how active we are each decade, we will see fantastic returns in our sixties. While some are looking forward to retirement, you will be living more fully than ever. These "golden years" are not necessarily a time to rest on your laurels and get ready for the home; they can and should be highly productive years that are tempered with just the right mixture of vigor and wisdom.

If you can maintain or increase your activity level in your seventies you will do much to ensure that you will remain self-sufficient, be less brittle, have a stronger immune system, be less susceptible to heart ailments and arterial problems, and be less likely to suffer from diseases. In your eighties, you don't have to miss a beat. You may consider reducing the intensity of your regular exercise, but our idol, Jack LaLanne, is a great testament to a healthy lifestyle, and although in his late eighties, he is as vital and energized as he was when he first entered our living rooms in the 1950s. If you can be active and nutritionally responsible through the time you are 85, you have a great shot at living to be 100.

Seen in this light, you can look at each stage of your life and value the quality rather than the quantity of those years, as you build a foundation for the years to come. After you have achieved your goal weight and eliminated excess body fat, you are equipped to live longer and have far greater health. Rather than putting on a pound or two every year, you can reduce body fat and increase your activity level. These lifestyle shifts that you have already made will see you through the rest of your years.

NOTES

1. J. O. Prochaska and C. C. DiClemente. *The Transtheoretical Approach: Crossing the Traditional Boundaries of Therapy*. Melbourne, Fla.: Krieger Publishing, 1984.
2. U.S. Department of Health and Human Services. *CDC's Guidelines for School and Community Programs: Promoting Lifelong Physical Activity*. National Centers for Disease Control and Prevention.
3. S. K. Power and S. C. Dodd. *Total Fitness: Exercise, Nutrition, and Wellness, 2nd ed.* Boston: Allyn and Bacon, 1999.
4. *Virginia Post Pilot,* 30 October 1995.
5. K. W. Cullen and T. Baronowski. "Influence of Family Dinner on Food Intake of 4th to 6th Grade Students." *Journal of American Dietetics*, Supplement 100 (September 2000). SUNY Buffalo. Nurses' Health Study II. Baylor College of Medicine.
6. U.S. Department of Agriculture. U.S. Department of Health and Human Services. U.S.D.A. Food Guide Pyramid 2000.
   http://www.pueblo.gsa.gov/cic = _text/food-pyramid/main.htm.
7. American Institute for Cancer Research. American Dietetic Association. Pendleton Methodist Memorial Hospital. The Nutrition Institute of Louisiana at Methodist Hospital. Dr. Albert Barracas, M.D., F.A.C.S.
8. L. K. Mahan and S. Escott-Stump. *Krause's Food, Nutrition, and Diet Therapy, 10th ed.* Philadelphia: D. B. Saunders, 2000.
9. Power and Dodd. *Total Fitness.*
10. W. D. McCardle, F. I. Katch, and V. L. Katch. *Exercise Physiology: Exercise, Nutrition, and Human Performance*. Philadelphia: Lea & Febiger, 1991.
11. Centers for Disease Control and Prevention, U.S. Department of Health and Human Services, U.S. Surgeon General's Report (1995). American Cancer Society. American Heart and Lung Association.
12. J. S. Greenberg and D. Pargman. *Physical Fitness: A Wellness Approach, 2nd ed.* Englewood Cliffs, N.J.: Prentice-Hall, 1989. F. I. Katch and W. D. McCardle. *Introduction to Nutrition, Exercise, and Health, 4th ed.* Philadelphia: Lea & Febiger, 1993.
13. Provided by Anne K. LeMay, M.A., M.F.C.C.
14. Provided by John Troop, Ph.D.

INDEX